AMOGS
Practical Manual of
Thyroid in Pregnancy

AMOGS
Practical Manual of
Thyroid in Pregnancy

Editor-in-Chief

Kiran Kurtkoti
MBBS DGO DFP DNB FICOG FMCOG
Obstetrician Gynecologist
President
Association of Maharashtra Obstetric and
Gynaecological Societies (AMOGS)
Director
Shashwat Multi-speciality Hospitals India Pvt. Ltd.
Pune, Maharashtra, India

Editor

Madhuri Mehendale
MBBS DGO FCPS DNB (OBGY) FICOG
Diploma in Advanced Laparoscopy and ART (Kiel, Germany)
Additional Associate Professor
Lokmanya Tilak Municipal Medical College
Mumbai, Maharashtra, India

JAYPEE

JAYPEE BROTHERS MEDICAL PUBLISHERS
The Health Sciences Publisher
New Delhi | London

JAYPEE **Jaypee Brothers Medical Publishers (P) Ltd**

Headquarters
EMCA House, 23/23-B
Ansari Road, Daryaganj
New Delhi 110 002, India
Landline: +91-11-23272143, +91-11-23272703
+91-11-23282021, +91-11-23245672
e-mail: jaypee@jaypeebrothers.com

Corporate Office
4838/24, Ansari Road, Daryaganj
New Delhi 110 002, India
Phone: +91-11-43574357
Fax: +91-11-43574314
e-mail: jaypee@jaypeebrothers.com

Overseas Office
JP Medical Ltd.
83, Victoria Street, London
SW1H 0HW (UK)
Phone: +44-20 3170 8910
e-mail: info@jpmedpub.com

EU GPSR Authorised Representative
Logos Europe, 9 rue Nicolas Poussin
17000, La Rochelle, France
Phone: +33 (0) 6 67 93 73 78
e-mail: contact@logoseurope.eu

Website: www.jaypeebrothers.com
Website: www.jaypeedigital.com

Inquiries for bulk sales may be solicited at: jaypee@jaypeebrothers.com

AMOGS Practical Manual of Thyroid in Pregnancy

First Edition: **2026**

ISBN: 978-93-7202-923-9

Printed at: Samrat Offset Pvt. Ltd.

Contributors

Aishwarya Agrawal
MBBS MS (OBGY) DNB (OBGY) PGDMLS
Fellow
Department of Fetal Medicine
ADI Advanced Centre for Fetal Care
Bengaluru, Karnataka, India

Kiran Kurtkoti
MBBS DGO DFP DNB FICOG FMCOG
Obstetrician Gynecologist
President
Association of Maharashtra Obstetric and Gynaecological Societies (AMOGS)
Director
Shashwat Multi-speciality Hospitals India Pvt. Ltd.
Pune, Maharashtra, India

Madhuri Mehendale
MBBS DGO FCPS DNB (OBGY) FICOG Diploma in Advanced Laparoscopy and ART (Kiel, Germany)
Additional Associate Professor
Lokmanya Tilak Municipal Medical College
Mumbai, Maharashtra, India

Meenal S Sarmalkar
MD (OBGY) DNB DGO DFP
Professor (Additional)
Department of Obstetrics and Gynecology
Lokmanya Tilak Municipal Medical College and General Hospital
Mumbai, Maharashtra, India

Nitin Kshirsagar MD DGO FICOG
Professor
Department of Obstetrics and Gynecology
Krishna Vishwa Vidyapeeth
Karad, Maharashtra, India

Payal C Rathod MS (OBGY)
Assistant Professor
Department of Obstetrics and Gynecology
Lokmanya Tilak Municipal Medical College and General Hospital
Mumbai, Maharashtra, India

Shraddha Joshi Shastri
DNB (OBGYN) DGO MBBS
Professor
Department of Obstetrics and Gynecology
Smt. Kashibai Navale Medical College
Pune, Maharashtra, India

Shweta Avinash Khade
MBBS DNB DGO FMAS FICOG Dip ART (Kiel, Germany)
Associate Professor—Additional
Department of Obstetrics and Gynecology
Lokmanya Tilak Municipal Medical College and General Hospital
Mumbai, Maharashtra, India

Smurti Kamble
MBBS MS FMAS Dip ART (Kiel, Germany)
Assistant Professor
Department of Obstetrics and Gynecology
Lokmanya Tilak Municipal Medical College and General Hospital
Mumbai, Maharashtra, India

Srushti S Joshi MBBS MS DNB FRM
Consultant Fertility Specialist
RheumaGyn Clinic
Mumbai, Maharashtra, India

Uma Wankhede MBBS MD (OBGY)
Professor and Head
Department of Obstetrics and Gynecology
Government Medical College (GMC)
Pune, Maharashtra, India

Vaishali Korde-Nayak
MBBS DGO DNB MNAMS FICOG Fellow Maternal and Fetal Medicine, NUH Singapore
Professor and Head
Department of Obstetrics and Gynecology
MIMER Medical College, Pune
Senior Critical Care Consultant
Ruby Hall Clinic
Pune, Maharashtra, India

Vijaya Deepthi M MBBS MS (OBGYN)
Assistant Professor
Department of Obstetrics and Gynecology
Smt. Kashibai Navale Medical College
Pune, Maharashtra, India

Zubin Sheriar MS (OBGY)
Consultant
Department of Obstetrics and Gynecology
Aviva Clinic for Women
Mumbai, Maharashtra, India

Preface

Thyroid function is fundamental to maternal and fetal well-being, and disturbances in its regulation remain a significant cause of pregnancy-related complications. Advances in endocrinology and obstetric care have deepened our understanding of thyroid physiology in pregnancy, allowing clinicians to diagnose and manage disorders with greater precision, safety, and sensitivity to maternal needs.

This book offers a comprehensive yet practical exploration of thyroid health during pregnancy. It brings together essential scientific foundations with real-world clinical applications, covering core topics such as the *basics of thyroid physiology, normal adaptive changes in pregnancy,* and the nuanced management of *hyperthyroidism, hypothyroidism,* and *postpartum thyroiditis*. Each chapter is designed to provide clear, evidence-based guidance that supports accurate assessment, timely intervention, and prevention of complications. Special emphasis is placed on individualized care, recognizing the diversity of presentations and the importance of tailored therapeutic approaches.

Our goal is not only to inform but also to encourage thoughtful, ethical, and compassionate practice in the care of pregnant women with thyroid disorders. By simplifying complex concepts and presenting them with clinical clarity, we hope this book serves as both a trusted reference and a supportive companion in decision-making.

Ultimately, understanding thyroid function in pregnancy extends beyond medical management—it safeguards the health, confidence, and future of mothers and their babies. It is our sincere hope that this work contributes meaningfully to that mission.

Kiran Kurtkoti
Madhuri Mehendale

Acknowledgments

It is with great pride and heartfelt appreciation that we present the *AMOGS Practical Manual of Thyroid in Pregnancy*—a collaborative academic achievement that embodies the vision and unwavering commitment of the Association of Maharashtra Obstetric and Gynaecological Societies (AMOGS) and the Maharashtra College of Obstetricians and Gynaecologists (MCOG).

We express our sincere gratitude to the AMOGS Office Bearers for their enduring encouragement and steadfast support. Their belief in this initiative has provided both direction and inspiration throughout its development. Our thanks extend to all AMOGS members, whose enthusiasm for academic advancement and excellence in clinical care continues to elevate our collective work.

A special note of appreciation goes to the authors and contributors who generously dedicated their time and shared their extensive expertise. Their evidence-based, insightful, and practically relevant chapters form the backbone of this manual and significantly enrich its value for clinicians. We are equally grateful to the reviewers, mentors, and colleagues whose thoughtful feedback strengthened the clarity and rigor of this publication.

We express our sincere appreciation to the team at M/s Jaypee Brothers Medical Publishers (P) Ltd, New Delhi, India, for their outstanding support and professionalism. In particular, we thank Shri Jitendar P Vij (Group Chairman), Mr Ankit Vij (Managing Director), Ms Pooja Bhandari [Director-Production (Books and Journals)], Mr Sabyasachi Hazra (Director, PG and PNR Content), and Mr Akhilesh Saxena (Development Editor) for their tremendous efforts in bringing this book to fruition.

On behalf of AMOGS, we dedicate this manual to clinicians, postgraduate students, and learners committed to advancing women's health through informed and compassionate fertility care.

With warm regards and deep gratitude.

Kiran Kurtkoti
Madhuri Mehendale

Acknowledgements

Contents

CHAPTER 1

Understanding Basics of Thyroid

Meenal S Sarmalkar, Payal C Rathod

INTRODUCTION

The thyroid gland is a highly vascular and butterfly-shaped endocrine gland located in the anterior neck. Despite its small size, it plays a pivotal role in regulating metabolism, thermogenesis, growth, and overall physiological balance through the secretion of thyroid hormones.[1-5] Its detailed structure and precisely regulated function make it one of the most important endocrine organs.

GROSS ANATOMY OF THE THYROID GLAND

The thyroid lies anterior to the trachea and inferior to the larynx, extending from C5 to T1 vertebrae. It consists of two lateral lobes connected by an isthmus across the second to third tracheal rings.[6] A pyramidal lobe may extend superiorly as a remnant of the thyroglossal duct.[6,7] The overall gross morphology is illustrated in **Figure 1**.[8]

Each lobe typically measures 4–6 cm in length and 1–3 cm in thickness. In adults, the gland weighs approximately 15–20 g, although size varies with iodine intake and hormonal stimulation.[1]

MICROSCOPIC STRUCTURE

Histologically, the thyroid is composed of numerous spherical follicles lined by cuboidal follicular cells and filled with colloid, which contains

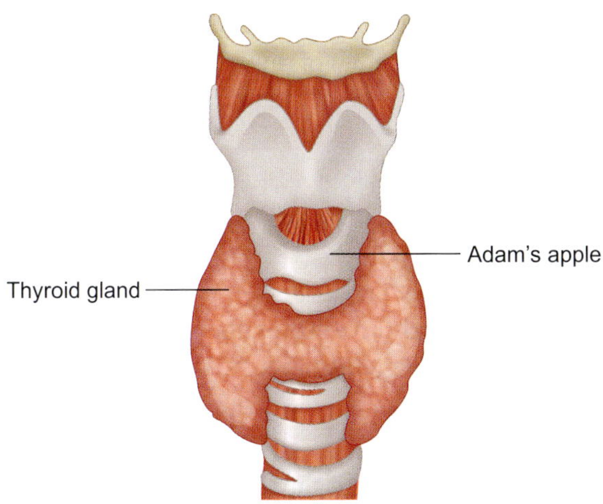

Fig. 1: Gross anatomy of thyroid gland.[8]

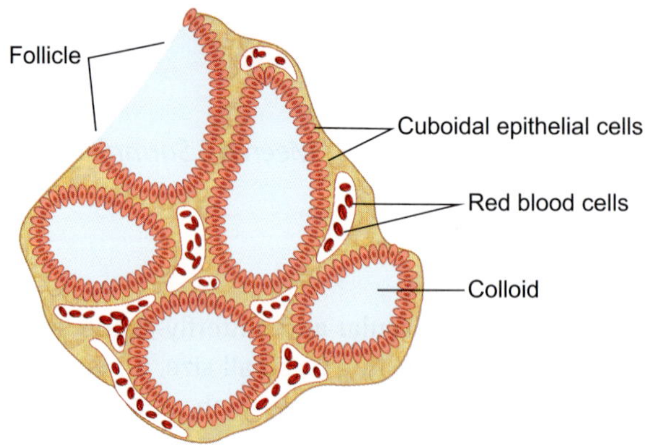

Fig. 2: Microscopic structure of thyroid gland.[8]

thyroglobulin—the precursor of T3 and T4.[1] This microscopic architecture is shown in **Figure 2**. Parafollicular (C) cells located between follicles secrete calcitonin, which helps to regulate serum calcium levels.[7]

EMBRYOLOGICAL DEVELOPMENT

The thyroid gland develops from the thyroid diverticulum arising from the primitive pharynx. It migrates downward via the thyroglossal duct, which normally involutes. Failure of regression may result in thyroglossal cysts or ectopic thyroid tissue.[6]

BLOOD SUPPLY, VENOUS DRAINAGE, NERVE SUPPLY, AND LYMPHATICS

The extensive vascularity of the gland is depicted in **Figure 3**.

Arterial Supply

- Superior thyroid artery—branch of the external carotid artery
- Inferior thyroid artery—branch of the thyrocervical trunk[6]

Venous Drainage

- Superior thyroid vein
- Middle thyroid vein
- Inferior thyroid vein[6]

The gland receives nearly five times its weight in blood per minute, reflecting its high metabolic activity.[1]

Nerve Supply

- Sympathetic fibers from cervical ganglia
- Parasympathetic fibers from the vagus nerve[6]

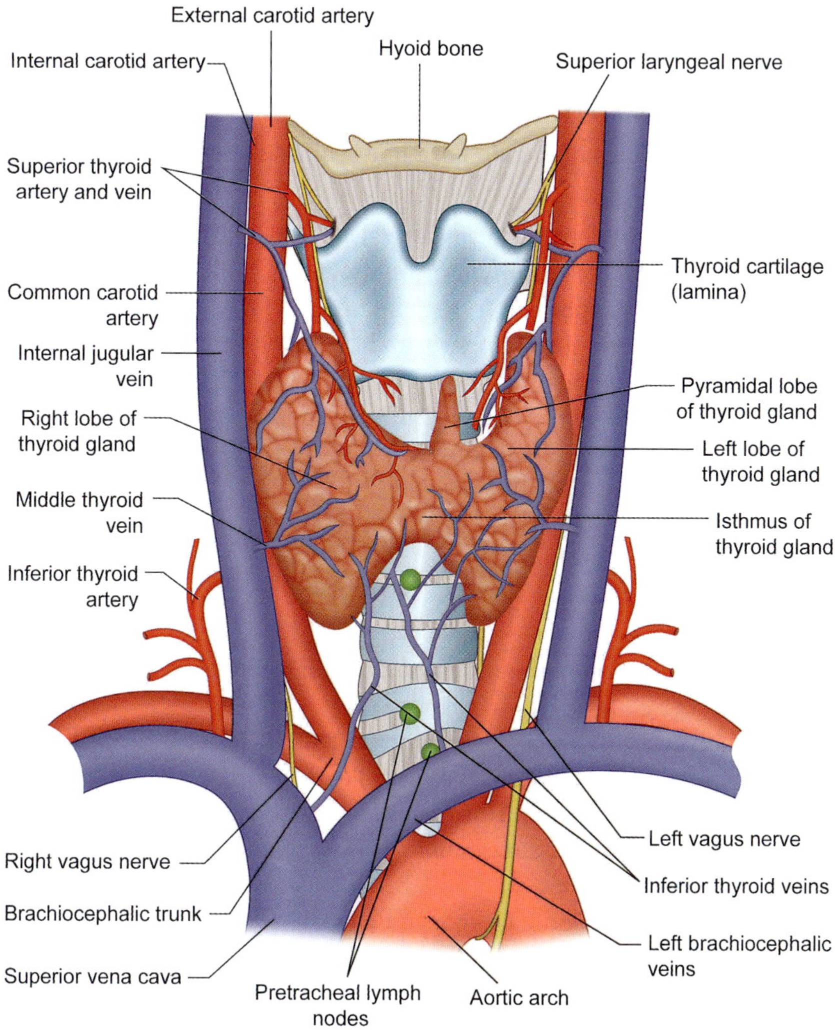

Fig. 3: Blood supply of thyroid gland.[6]

Lymphatics

Drain into prelaryngeal, pretracheal, and paratracheal nodes, then into deep cervical lymph nodes.[6]

IODINE METABOLISM AND PHYSIOLOGY OF THYROID HORMONES

Dietary iodine is absorbed in the intestine and transported to the thyroid under thyroid stimulating hormone (TSH) stimulation. Within the follicles, it integrates into thyroglobulin to form T3 and T4.[2] Approximately 80% of circulating T3 is produced by peripheral conversion of T4, and T3 is 3–5 times more potent.[3]

SYNTHESIS OF THYROID HORMONES (T3 AND T4)

The biochemical steps of thyroid hormone synthesis are shown in **Figure 4** and include:[3]

Thyroid hormone synthesis involves several coordinated steps:

1. *Iodide uptake (iodide trapping):* Iodide enters follicular cells via the sodium-iodide symporter (NIS), stimulated by TSH.
2. *Oxidation of iodide:* Thyroid peroxidase (TPO) catalyses conversion of iodide to active iodine.
3. *Iodination of tyrosine (Organification):* Iodine attaches to tyrosine residues on thyroglobulin to form:
   - Monoiodotyrosine (MIT)
   - Diiodotyrosine (DIT)
4. *Coupling reaction:*
   - DIT + DIT → T4
   - MIT + DIT → T3
5. *Storage:* The hormone-bound thyroglobulin is stored as colloid within follicles.
6. *Endocytosis and proteolysis:* Under TSH stimulation, colloid is endocytosed and proteolytically cleaved to release T3 and T4.
7. *Secretion into circulation:* Hormones enter bloodstream predominantly bound to thyroxine-binding globulin (TBG), albumin, and transthyretin.
8. *Peripheral conversion:*
   - Types 1 and 2 deiodinases convert T4 → T3
   - Type 3 deiodinase converts T4 → rT3 (inactive)

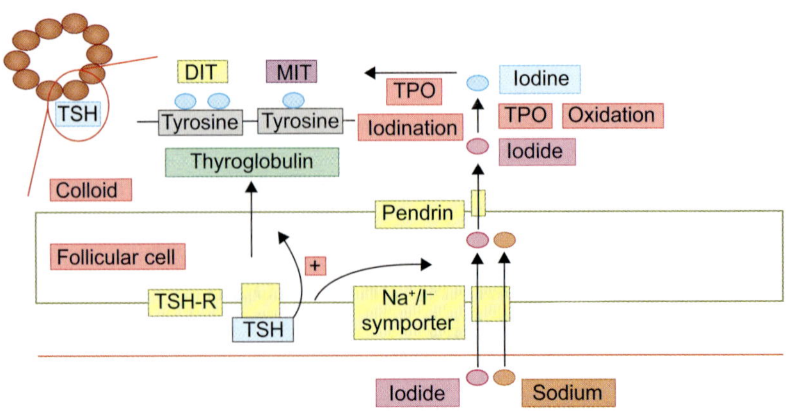

Fig. 4: Thyroid hormone synthesis.[7]

REGULATION OF THYROID FUNCTION

Regulation occurs via the hypothalamic-pituitary-thyroid (HPT) axis, illustrated in **Figure 5**. The HPT axis maintains hormonal balance:

- Hypothalamus releases TRH → stimulates pituitary
- Pituitary secretes TSH → stimulates thyroid
- Rising T3 and T4 exert negative feedback on both TRH and TSH[2]

Additional regulators:

- *Inhibitors:* Somatostatin, glucocorticoids, and dopamine
- Thyrotropin-releasing hormone (TRH) also stimulates prolactin release.

PHYSIOLOGICAL ROLES OF THYROID HORMONES

Metabolic Effects

- Increases glucose absorption.
- Enhances gluconeogenesis.
- Promotes lipolysis.
- Increases protein turnover → may result in net protein loss.
- Produces a negative nitrogen balance.[4]

Cardiovascular System

T3 increases cardiac output, heart rate, and contractility while reducing systemic vascular resistance.[4]

Sympathetic Nervous System

T3 upregulates β-adrenergic receptors in cardiac muscle, skeletal muscle, and adipose tissues.[4]

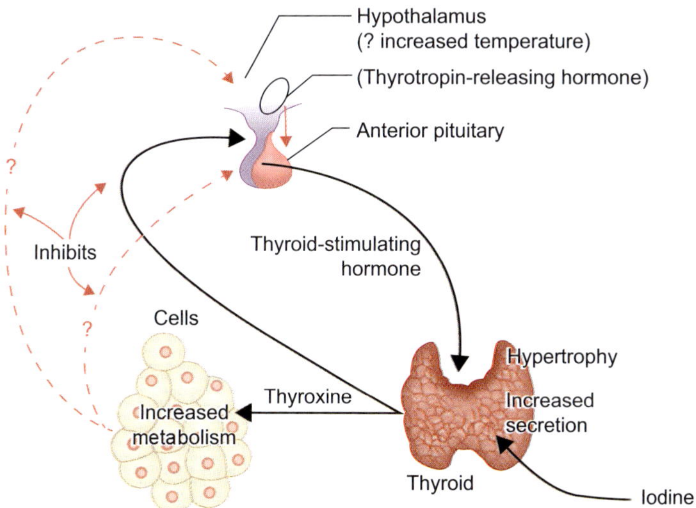

Fig. 5: Regulation of thyroid function.[8]

Diagnostic Evaluation of Thyroid Disorders

- *Laboratory tests:* TSH, free T3, and free T4
- *Imaging:* Thyroid ultrasound and radionuclide scan
- Autoantibodies: Anti-TPO, anti-TG, and TSH receptor antibodies[1,4]

THYROID DISORDERS

Hypothyroidism

A deficiency of thyroid hormone results in fatigue, weight gain, cold intolerance, menstrual disturbances, and metabolic slowing.[5]

Types

- *Primary overt hypothyroidism:* ↓T3/T4, ↑TSH
- *Subclinical hypothyroidism:* Normal T3/T4, ↑TSH
- *Secondary hypothyroidism:* ↓T3/T4, ↓TSH[5] (pituitary/hypothalamic disease)

Common Causes

- Iodine deficiency
- Hashimoto's thyroiditis
- Radioiodine ablation
- Thyroidectomy
- *Drugs:* Lithium and amiodarone[5]

Reproductive Effects

Hypothyroidism reduces sex hormone-binding globulin (SHBG) and alters estrogen/testosterone balance, leading to oligomenorrhea, menorrhagia, or amenorrhea.[5] Ovulatory dysfunction contributes to subfertility, especially in overt hypothyroidism.

Management in women seeking conception—TSH should be maintained below the 1st-trimester upper normal limit.[5]

Hyperthyroidism

Characterized by excess circulating thyroid hormones causing weight loss, heat intolerance, tremors, anxiety, and tachycardia.[4]

Types

- *Overt hyperthyroidism:* ↑T3/T4, ↓TSH
- *Subclinical hyperthyroidism:* Normal T3/T4, ↓TSH
- *Secondary hyperthyroidism:* ↑T3/T4, ↑TSH (rare)[4]

Common Causes

- Graves' disease
- Toxic multinodular goiter[4]

Reproductive Effects

Menstrual irregularities may include oligomenorrhea or amenorrhea, though ovulatory disturbance is less pronounced than in hypothyroidism.[4]

CONCLUSION

The thyroid gland, though small in size, exerts profound effects on metabolism, cardiovascular function, neurological activity, and reproductive health through the tightly regulated synthesis and secretion of thyroid hormones. An understanding of its anatomy, histology, embryological development, vascular supply, and physiological mechanisms provides the foundation for comprehending both normal thyroid function and disease states. Precise regulation via the hypothalamic-pituitary-thyroid axis ensures hormonal homeostasis, while disturbances at any level of this axis can result in clinically significant hypo- or hyperthyroidism. Given the wide-ranging systemic and reproductive consequences of thyroid dysfunction—particularly in women of reproductive age—early diagnosis, appropriate evaluation, and timely management are essential. A comprehensive grasp of thyroid structure and function is therefore critical for effective clinical assessment and therapeutic decision-making in endocrine and reproductive medicine.

REFERENCES

1. Larsen PR, Kronenberg HM. Williams Textbook of Endocrinology, 13th edition. Philadelphia, PA: Elsevier; 2016. pp. 333-68.
2. Brent GA. Mechanisms of thyroid hormone action. In: Melmed S, Polonsky KS, Reed Larsen P, Kronenberg HM (Eds). Williams Textbook of Endocrinology, 13th edition. Philadelphia, PA: Elsevier; 2016. pp. 292-312.
3. Kopp P. Thyroid hormone synthesis. In: Melmed S, Polonsky KS, Reed Larsen P, Kronenberg HM (Eds). Williams Textbook of Endocrinology, 13th edition. Philadelphia, PA: Elsevier; 2016. pp. 313-32.
4. Cooper DS. Hyperthyroidism. In: Melmed S, Polonsky KS, Reed Larsen P, Kronenberg HM (Eds). Williams Textbook of Endocrinology, 13th edition. Philadelphia, PA: Elsevier; 2016. pp. 369-94.
5. Brent GA. Hypothyroidism and thyroiditis. In: Melmed S, Polonsky KS, Reed Larsen P, Kronenberg HM (Eds). Williams Textbook of Endocrinology, 13th edition. Philadelphia, PA: Elsevier; 2016. pp. 395-420.
6. Standring S. Gray's Anatomy: The Anatomical Basis of Clinical Practice, 40th edition. Philadelphia, PA: Elsevier; 2008. pp. 462-4.
7. Barrett KE, Barman SM, Brooks HL, Yuan JXJ. Ganong's Review of Medical Physiology, 26th edition. United States: McGraw-Hill; 2019. p. 318.
8. Hall JE. Guyton and Hall Textbook of Medical Physiology, 13th edition. Philadelphia, PA: Elsevier; 2015. pp. 932-9.

CHAPTER 2

Physiological Changes in Thyroid Function during Pregnancy

Shraddha Joshi Shastri, Vijaya Deepthi M

INTRODUCTION

The prevalence of thyroid disorders in pregnant women in the Indian Subcontinent is high with some studies showing 33.9%.[1] After Diabetes, they are the most common endocrine disorder found in pregnant women. A 2021 meta-analysis of observational studies in India found the pooled prevalence of hypothyroidism to be 11.07%, subclinical hypothyroidism being the most common accounting for 9.51%.[2] Prevalence is more in inland areas as opposed to coastal areas probably due to iodine deficiency. Also, a varied prevalence is noted in the different ethnic groups that are seen in India. Hyperthyroidism is rarer with some studies showing a prevalence of 2.3%. As the fetus is dependent completely on maternal thyroxin, free T4 in the 1st trimester, untreated hypothyroidism can lead to suboptimal IQ and learning difficulties in academics. Other complications of untreated hypothyroidism include miscarriage, premature birth, growth restricted fetus, stillbirths.[3] Thyroid disorders are usually preexisting but can develop after conception. It is important for clinicians to detect thyroid disorders preconceptionally or early on in pregnancy and treat adequately to prevent the said complications.

Thyroid disorders may be seen as an increase in size of the thyroid gland or a change in level of thyroid hormones or the presence of autoantibodies that are developed that affect the mother as well as the fetus and the neonate once born. Hence, it is important to understand the physiology of the thyroid gland in pregnancy for the correct interpretation of the thyroid function tests in the various trimesters of pregnancy.[4]

NORMAL PHYSIOLOGIC CHANGES IN PREGNANCY

The state of pregnancy witnesses significant changes in size and function of the thyroid gland. Nearing term, the thyroid gland increases by almost a third in size. The increase in the size of thyroid gland is mainly due to hyperplasia and increased vascularity. Within the thyroid follicle, iodide is organified onto tyrosine residues in thyroglobulin to generate mono- and di-iodotyrosine, which couple to form T4, and to a lesser extent, T3. Most circulating thyroid hormone is T4, and it is largely protein-bound, mainly to thyroxine-binding globulin (TBG), others being thyroxine binding prealbumin or transthyretin, and albumin. Positive feedback from the thyroid-stimulating hormone (TSH) from anterior pituitary as it stimulates the thyroid epithelial receptors, increases the production and release of thyroxine **(Fig. 1)**.

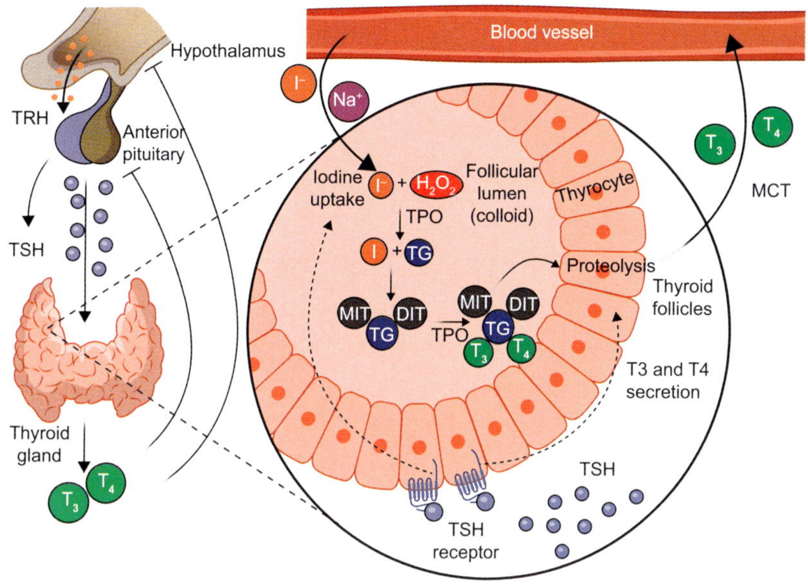

Fig. 1: Depicting normal production of thyroid hormones. (MCT: monocarboxylate transporter; TG: thyroglobulin; TRH: thyrotropin-releasing hormone; TSH: thyroid-stimulating hormone)

Pregnancy is a state of increased metabolism, catering to a growing fetus which has its own metabolism. Hence, the size of thyroid gland increases and iodine uptake also increases. However, pregnancy is a euthyroid state. Hence, in spite of an increase in thyroid activity, the levels of TSH, free T4 and free T3 remain within the normal range.

Human chorionic gonadotropin (hCG) and chorionic thyrotropin are secreted by the placenta and they act on the thyroid and stimulate it.[5] This is due to similar molecular structure of α-hCG and TSH, and their respective receptors being similar. Toward the end of the 3rd month of pregnancy in humans, when hCG levels are highest, it causes significant thyroid-stimulation along with TSH.[6] During this time, blood levels of TSH often are suppressed. In conditions like molar pregnancy, hCG-secreting tumors, multiple pregnancies where hCG levels are very elevated, the thyrotropic activity is so much that it could cause clinical hyperthyroidism.

EFFECT OF HUMAN CHORIONIC GONADOTROPIN

As described by Glinoer D et al.,[7] TSH and α-component of hCG are similar. Their receptors are similar. Hence, hCG can bind to the TSH receptor on thyroid epithelial cells. As a result, it causes:

- Increased thyroxine production, free T4 levels in the 1st trimester
- Slight reduction in serum TSH levels in the 1st trimester **(Fig. 2)**

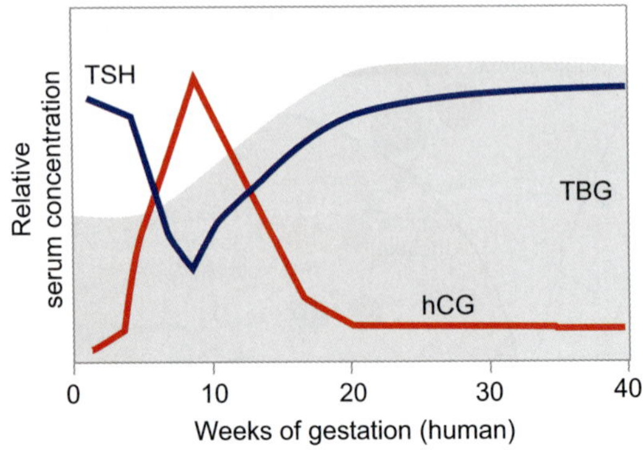

Fig. 2: Levels of human chorionic gonadotropin (hCG) against the gestational age of the fetus. (TBG: thyroxine-binding globulin; TSH: thyroid-stimulating hormone)

- Slight increase in the TSH levels in the 2nd trimester. TSH levels increase further in the 3rd trimester.

Hence, we require trimester cut-offs while interpreting TSH levels. Also, TSH values vary greatly with respect to the geographic location and ethnicity of the population.

Pregnancy, therefore, is a hypermetabolic state with increased demand on the thyroid gland. This, however, does not appear to affect normal individuals but in women with subclinical hypothyroidism, this extra demand in pregnancy can setup clinical disease.

EFFECT OF ESTROGEN ON THYROID-BINDING GLOBULIN

The main serum protein that transports thyroid hormones in blood is the TBG. It is the protein with the highest affinity for T4 (thyroxine). Estrogen stimulates increased production of binding proteins in the liver. The normal rise of estrogen levels during pregnancy is such that there is roughly a doubling in serum TBG concentrations. Rise in levels of TBG binds with free T4 and leads to lowered free T4 concentrations. Consequently, enhanced production of TSH by the anterior pituitary induces a rise in secretion of thyroid hormones. A new physiological equilibrium is noted between free and bound thyroid hormones and, thus, a significant increase in total T4 and T3 levels. The demand remains stable till term. Hence, there is a rise in total T3 and T4 levels. Free T3 and T4 levels are either normal or in the upper limits of normal. It is, therefore, recommended to check both serum TSH and unbound hormone levels. In usual practice, free T3 levels are not used. So, serum TSH and free T4 levels are used to evaluate thyroid function **(Fig. 3)**.

IODINE METABOLISM

The requirement of iodine increases from 150 to 250 µg/day during pregnancy. This is due to:

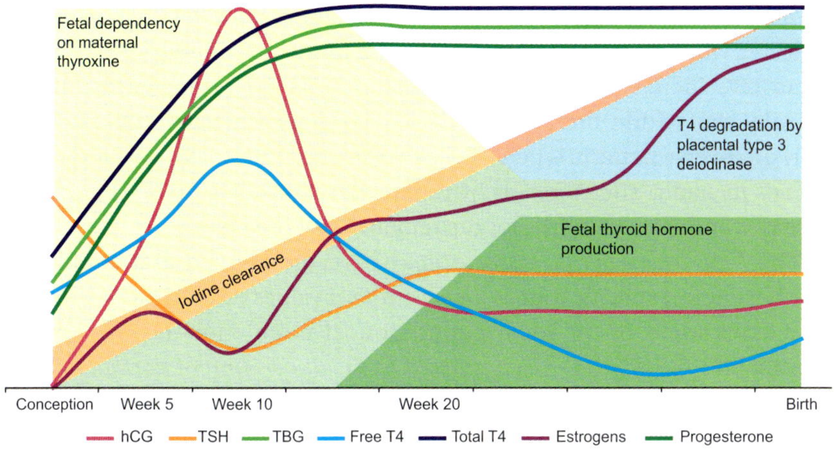

Fig. 3: Levels of various hormones against the gestational age of the fetus.

- Increased secretion of thyroid hormone by thyroid gland to maintain euthyroid status
- Increased renal iodine clearance
- Fetal iodine requirements

In inland areas with even mild or moderate iodine deficiency, gradual decrease in iodine stores is noted from the 1st to 3rd trimesters. Hence, pregnant women are advised to consume only iodized salt as India is one of the countries with areas of iodine deficiency. *Increasing iodine intake from the standard 100–150 μg/day to at least 200 μg/day during pregnancy is recommended by the World Health Organization.*

PLACENTAL TRANSFER OF THYROID HORMONES

As described by Calvo RM et al. (2002),[8] free T4 from the maternal circulation crosses the placenta and is the main source of thyroxine for the fetal brain development till 12 weeks of gestation until the fetal thyroid secretes hormones of its own. Maternal serum TSH does not cross the placenta; however, the TSH receptor stimulating and inhibiting hormones do cross the placenta and cause fetal hyper- or hypothyroidism, respectively. Maternal serum freely crosses the placenta and are taken up by the fetus. Hence, maternal iodine levels are critical for optimal fetal thyroid function. Radioactive iodine treatments are, hence, contraindicated in pregnancy as they enter fetal circulation and cause fetal thyroid ablation. Antithyroid drugs cross the placenta and suppress fetal thyroid function.

Thyroid Function Tests during Pregnancy

Serum TBG concentrations rise rapidly in early gestation and reach a plateau of roughly twice the nonpregnant level by around 15 weeks, remaining elevated for the rest of pregnancy. Total T4 shows a modest rise in the 1st trimester, whereas total T3 tends to increase more prominently.

As TBG increases, the free fractions of T4 and T3 transiently fall, but typically stay within the normal reference range. Maternal hCG and TSH show an inverse pattern: when hCG peaks at about 10 weeks' gestation, TSH reaches its nadir. Thereafter, as hCG concentrations decline, TSH gradually increases and then stabilizes for the remainder of pregnancy.

The *American Thyroid Association* has recommended that population based, trimester specific ranges for serum TSH values need to be ascertained after assessment of the local population. If population-specific data is unavailable, *4 μIU/mL to be considered as the upper limit of normal for TSH in pregnancy.*

Ministry of Health and Family Welfare, Govt. of India (2014), recommends *2.5 μIU/mL in the 1st trimester, 3 μIU/mL as the cutoff for TSH levels in the second and the third trimester.* These levels are based off of American Thyroid Association guidelines.[9]

As described by Tsuruta E et al.,[10] many of the pregnant women with hyperemesis gravidarum have thyroid profile laboratory values depicting hyperthyroidism. Higher levels of hCG are noted in these women and the severity of hyperemesis is directly related to the degree of hyperthyroidism, due to thyrotropic activity of the hCG. These clinical manifestations may be linked to a specific subpopulation of hCG molecules, specifically, hCG with reduced sialic acid content, having greater thyrotropic bioactivity. Treatment with antithyroid medication is recommended, if the symptoms of hyperthyroidism are supported by appropriate laboratory values.

PHYSIOLOGY OF THYROID IN THE FETUS AND THE NEONATE

Between 8 and 10 weeks of gestation, the human fetal thyroid gland develops the capacity to concentrate iodine and synthesize hormone at the same time that the pituitary begins to synthesize TSH. Fetus concentrates iodine and fetal thyroid starts producing thyroid hormones from 12 weeks onward. Until then maternal thyroxine is the main source for the fetal neurological development. Terminal stages of brain differentiation, including synaptogenesis, growth of dendrites and axons, myelination and neuronal migration seem to be profoundly affected by the presence of optimal levels of maternal thyroxin.[11]

In the absence of the pituitary gland, some thyroid development and hormone synthesis is possible but optimal function requires TSH. Development of the pituitary-thyroid axis is completed by 12–14 weeks. Significant increase in fetal TSH is paramount until 20 weeks for proper functioning of the axis independent of maternal thyroxin. As with gonadotropins and other pituitary hormones, the rise in fetal thyroid activity parallels maturation of the hypothalamus and the establishment of the hypothalamic–pituitary portal circulation, which allows hypothalamic releasing hormones to reach the fetal pituitary. Fetal TSH concentrations increase and then level off around 28 weeks' gestation, remaining relatively high until delivery. Free T4 values climb steadily throughout this period, and by term, fetal T4 concentrations are higher than those of the mother **(Fig. 4)**. This pattern indicates a relative state of thyroidal hyperactivity in the fetus near term.[12]

During fetal life, T4 is the principal thyroid hormone produced, whereas both total and free T3 remain relatively low across gestation. In contrast, concentrations of reverse T3 (rT3) are high and tend to rise in parallel with T4. Most rT3 is generated by peripheral conversion of T4.[13] This pattern means that much of the fetal T4 pool is rapidly inactivated to rT3, which helps to limit energy expenditure and conserve substrates. At the cellular level, fetal thyroid hormones exert their effects by binding to nuclear thyroid hormone receptors and regulating the transcription of target genes.

Thyroid hormone receptors are widely distributed in the fetal brain, and present prior to the time the fetus is able to synthesize thyroid hormones.

Before the fetal thyroid gland becomes active, that is in the early weeks of pregnancy, the fetal brain is dependent on the placental transport of maternal T4. Hence, both overt and subclinical maternal hypothyroidism are associated with increased risks of miscarriage, preeclampsia, low birth weight, preterm delivery, and a decrease in IQ in the children.

Soon after birth, serum TSH concentrations increase rapidly to a peak at 30 minutes of age. They fall to baseline values by 48–72 hours. In response to this increase in TSH, total T4 and free T4 increase to peak values

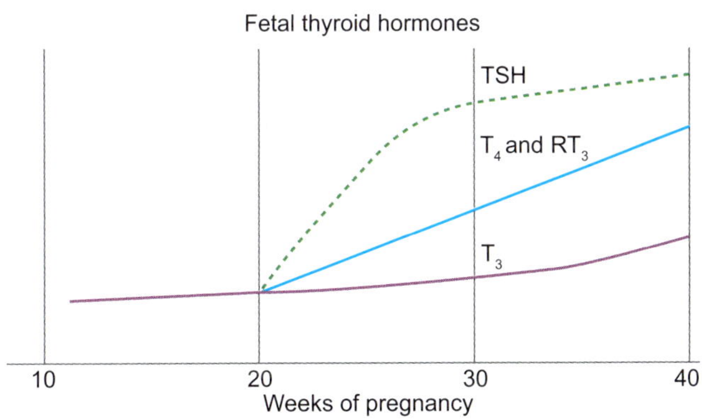

Relationship of weeks of pregnancy with fetal thyroid hormone levels

Fig. 4: Fetal thyroid-stimulating hormone (TSH) rises and reaches a plateau around 28 weeks of pregnancy. Free T4 concentration increases progressively, reaching adult levels near term. T4 is the major thyroid hormone secreted by the fetus.

by 24–48 hours of age. T3 levels increase even more, peaking by 24 hours of life. By 3–4 weeks of life, the thyroidal hyperactivity disappears. The postnatal rise in TSH is associated with a prolactin rise, suggesting that both are increased in response to TRH. The TRH surge is thought to be a response to rapid neonatal cooling.

CONCLUSION

Thyroid physiology undergoes profound and predictable adaptations during pregnancy to meet the metabolic demands of the mother and the developing fetus. These changes, driven primarily by rising levels of hCG, estrogen-induced increases in TBG, and enhanced iodine requirements, result in altered thyroid function tests that necessitate trimester- and population-specific reference ranges for accurate interpretation. Pregnancy itself remains a euthyroid state; however, women with limited thyroid reserve or pre-existing thyroid dysfunction may decompensate, leading to clinically significant disease.

Maternal thyroxine plays a critical role in early fetal neurodevelopment, particularly in the 1st trimester before the fetal thyroid becomes functional. Both overt and subclinical maternal hypothyroidism are, therefore, associated with adverse obstetric outcomes and long-term neurocognitive effects in the offspring. Adequate iodine intake, early identification of thyroid dysfunction, and appropriate monitoring are essential to ensure optimal maternal and fetal outcomes.

A clear understanding of the dynamic interplay between maternal, placental, and fetal thyroid physiology is fundamental for clinicians caring for pregnant women. Accurate interpretation of thyroid function tests, awareness of regional and ethnic variations, and timely intervention can significantly reduce preventable complications, underscoring the importance of thyroid health as an integral component of comprehensive antenatal care.

REFERENCES

1. Kumar R, Bansal R, Shergill HK, Garg P. Prevalence of thyroid dysfunction in pregnancy and its association with feto-maternal outcomes: A prospective observational study from a tertiary care institute in Northern India. Clin Epidemiol Global Health. 2023;19:101201.
2. Rajput R, Bajaj S, Ghosh S. Thyroid disorders in pregnancy: Consensus statement of Indian Thyroid Society. Off J Indian Thyroid Soc. 2023.
3. Davis LE, Leveno KL, Cunningham FG. Hypothyroidism complicating pregnancy. Obstet Gynecol. 1988;72(1):108-12.
4. Dashe JS, Casey BM, Wells CE, McIntire DD, Byrd EW, Leveno KJ, et al. Thyroid stimulating hormone in singleton and twin pregnancy: importance of gestational age-specific ranges. Obstet Gynecol. 2006;106:753.
5. Kennedy RL, Darne J. The role of hCG in regulation of the thyroid gland in normal and abnormal pregnancy. Obstet Gynecol. 1991;78:298.

6. Kimura M, Amino N, Tamaki H, Mitsuda N, Miyai K, Tanizawa O. Physiologic thyroid activation in normal early pregnancy is induced by circulating hCG. Obstet Gynecol. 1990;75:775.
7. Glinoer D, DeNayer P, Bourdoux P, Lemone M, Robyn C, Van Steirteghem A, et al. Regulation of maternal thyroid during pregnancy. J Clin Endocrinol Metab. 1990;71:276.
8. Calvo RM, Jauniaux E, Gulbis B, Asuncion M, Gervy C, Contempre B, et al. Fetal tissues are exposed to biologically relevant free thyroxine concentrations during early phases of development. J Clin Endocrinol Metab. 2002;87:1768.
9. Stagnaro-Green A, Abalovich M, Alexander E, Azizi F, Mestman J, Negro R, et al. Guidelines of the American Thyroid Association for the diagnosis and management of thyroid disease during pregnancy and postpartum. Thyroid. 2011;21:1081.
10. Tsuruta E, Tada H, Tamaki H, Kashiwai T, Asahio K, Takeoka K, et al. Pathogenic role of human chorionic gonadotropin in gestational thyrotoxicosis. J Clin Endocrinol Metab. 1995;80:350-5.
11. Leonard JL. Non-genomic actions of thyroid hormone in brain development. Steroids. 2008;73:1008-12.
12. Hume R, Simpson JL, Delahunty C, van Toor H, Wu SY, Williams FL, et al.; Scottish Preterm Thyroid Group. Human fetal and cord serum thyroid hormones: developmental trends and interrelationships. J Clin Endocrinol Metab. 2004;89:4097.
13. Thorpe-Beeston JG, Nicolaides KH, McGregor AM. Fetal thyroid function. Thyroid Thyroid. 1992;2(3):207-17.

CHAPTER 3

Hyperthyroidism in Pregnancy

Nitin Kshirsagar

INTRODUCTION

Thyroid dysfunction during pregnancy has profound impact on pregnant lady, fetus, and neonate. Physiological changes of pregnancy will alter the function of thyroid gland. Thyroid diseases may account for a number of complications. Interpretation of thyroid function tests is also different. Hence, it is imperative that obstetrician managing such cases should have fundamental knowledge of effect of pregnancy on thyroid function/ dysfunction and effects of thyroid diseases on pregnancy.

The subject is so important that the month of January is declared as "Thyroid awareness month".

In this article, let us review "Hyperthyroidism in Pregnancy".

Learning objectives:

- To define "Hyperthyroidism in pregnancy"
- To diagnose "Hyperthyroidism during pregnancy"
- To classify related hyperthyroid states
- To understand complications
- To plan the management
- To perform preconception counseling

DEFINITION OF HYPERTHYROIDISM

It is the condition in which thyroid gland is hyperactive and serum T4/T3 levels are more than the normal for that trimester serum thyroid-stimulating hormone (TSH) level is <0.1 μ/L.

Total T4/T3 values are more than one-and-half times raised above nonpregnant values.

In subclinical hyperthyroidism, TSH levels are <0.1while T4/T3 levels are normal.

PREVALENCE

- It is far less than hypothyroidism in pregnancy.
- It ranges from 0.1 to 1%.
- In India, it is <1%.

DIAGNOSIS OF HYPERTHYROIDISM

In most of the patients, clinical features are nonspecific.

Some symptoms due to physiological changes of pregnancy may mimic that of hyperthyroidism. Hence, the diagnosis is made by laboratory tests.

Common Symptoms

Heat intolerance, palpitations, anxiety, tremors, weight loss despite good appetite, dyspnea, excessive sweating, loose stools, vomiting, hyperactivity, and rapid speech.

Common Examination Findings

- Tachycardia (even during sleep)
- Irregular pulse (If atrial fibrillation)
- Tachypnea
- Systolic hypertension
- Warm and moist skin
- Thin and fine hair
- Proximal muscle weakness
- Exaggerated deep tendon reflexes
- Pretibial and/or periorbital edema
- Exophthalmos
- Goiter
- Exophthalmos, pretibial edema, and goiter are specific for Graves' disease.

Laboratory Diagnosis

Following investigations are advised for hyperthyroidism:

- Thyroid-stimulating hormone (total TSH or ultra TSH)
- T4 (total T4 or free T4)
- T3 (total T3 or free T3)

Thyrotropin Receptor Antibodies

Before interpreting thyroid function tests, one must remember how physiology of pregnancy alters these parameters:

- Higher levels of estrogen increase thyroid-binding globulin (TBG). Subsequently, total T4 and total T3 values are increased.
- Total T4 levels may increase up to one-and-half times that in nonpregnant state. So, when these levels are more than one-and-half times then only they are useful to diagnose hyperthyroidism in pregnancy.

However, free T4 and free T3 levels are unaffected. Hence, they are preferably used for confirming the diagnosis. Free T4 values are reliable if laboratory performs them by equilibrium dialysis or by ultrafiltration method. Immunoassay technique used by many laboratories for free T4 evaluation is not dependable.

Human chorionic gonadotropin (hCG) has structural similarities with TSH. During the 1st trimester when hCG secretion is highest in first 60–100 days of pregnancy, TSH is reduced significantly in about 15% cases.[1] Usually, it may be reduced to <0.1 μ/L. In extreme cases it may reach <0.01. After 16 weeks of gestation as the hCG level starts falling, TSH returns to normal level. Multiple pregnancy and smoking aggravate fall in TSH levels further.

Thyrotropin receptor antibodies may be reduced in 2nd and 3rd trimester of pregnancy. High levels of antibodies in late 3rd trimester may predict hyperthyroidism in neonate. In some cases, functional activity of antibodies against TSH receptors changes from stimulatory to inhibitory or blocking activity. These changes can affect laboratory parameters. It means thyroid function tests should be repeated frequently.

Thyrotropin antibodies should be assessed in following conditions:

- Pregnant lady with active hyperthyroidism
- History of treatment with radioactive iodine
- Prior thyroidectomy
- Previous neonate with hyperthyroidism

CLASSIFICATION OF HYPERTHYROIDISM DURING PREGNANCY

- Transient gestational thyrotoxicosis (TGT):
  - Hyperemesis gravidarum (HG)
  - Multiple pregnancy
  - Molar pregnancy
  - Hyperplacentosis
- Thyroid diseases:
  - Graves' disease
  - Thyroiditis
  - Multinodular goiter
- Iatrogenic:
  - Over treatment of hypothyroidism
  - Inadvertent intake of thyroid hormone (food contamination)

Gestational Transient Thyrotoxicosis

Definition: It is transient hyperthyroidism which is limited to first half of pregnancy and characterized by increased levels of T4 and suppressed or undetectable levels of TSH in the absence of thyrotropin antibodies.[2,3]

- Prevalence is 1–3% of pregnancies.
- Gestational transient thyrotoxicosis (GTT) is secondary to increased thyroid stimulation by hCG. It is observed in:
  - First trimester of pregnancy
  - Multiple pregnancy

- Vesicular mole
- Circulating hCG isoforms

Characteristics of GTT:

- Mild form and self-limiting
- No prior history of hyperthyroidism
- Resolves by early 2nd trimester of pregnancy
- By and large T3 and T4 levels are normal
- Ratio of T3/T4 is <20.
- Negative TRAb
- No goiter, no ophthalmopathy
- Blood flow on thyroid gland
- Doppler USG is not increased.

T4 levels are increased but T3 is normal or slightly elevated in 20% cases. There is peripheral conversion of T4 to inactive reverse T3 (rT3) due to starvation. Hence, T3/T4 ratio is <20.[4]

Hyperemesis Gravidarum

- The most common cause of TGT is HG.
- Prevalence is 0.5–10 per 1,000 pregnancies.[5]

Features of HG:

- Excessive vomiting
- Dehydration
- Electrolyte imbalance
- Ketonuria
- Weight loss by at least 5%
  - Confined to 1st trimester of pregnancy
  - Suppressed TSH levels and slightly increased levels of T4 are observed in 30–60% cases **(Table 1)**.

Graves' Disease

It is the most common form of hyperthyroidism. In 96% of the cases, it is due to TRAb. The prevalence is 0.1–1%. Prevalence of subclinical type is 0.6%. It is

TABLE 1: Differences between hyperemesis gravidarum (HG) and Graves' disease.

Features	*Graves' disease*	*HG*
Symptoms of hyperthyroidism before pregnancy	+	–
Nausea and vomiting	+	++
Goiter and ophthalmopathy	+	–
Thyrotropin receptor antibodies	++	–
T4 levels	↑↑↑	↑
Total T3/total T4 ratio	>20	<20

Flowchart 1: Complications.

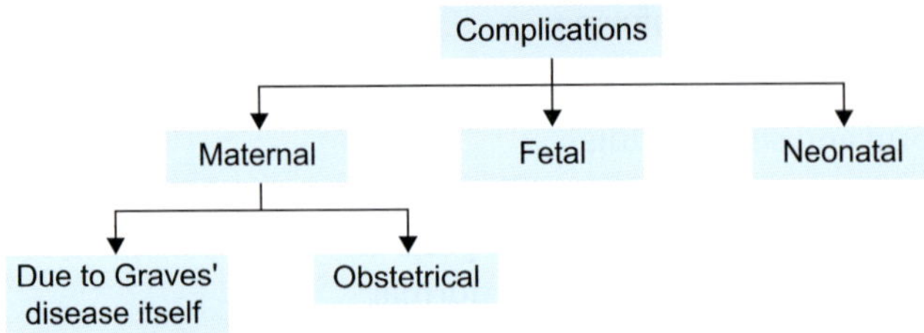

aggravated in 1st trimester of pregnancy, however, there can be amelioration later on beyond 2nd and 3rd trimester of pregnancy. Clinically, the patients will have typical symptoms of hyperthyroidism mentioned earlier.

Apart from the general signs like tachycardia (even during sleep), irregular pulse, etc., the hallmark of Graves' disease, ophthalmopathy, goiter, periorbital, and/or pretibial edema.

The diagnosis is confirmed by suppressed TSH and high T4 levels with presence of TRAb **(Flowchart 1)**.

THYROID STORM

- It is a life-threatening complication in whom hyperthyroidism is undiagnosed or uncontrolled.
- Prevalence is 2.7/100,000 pregnancies.[6]
- Precipitating factors are labor, surgery, infection, and trauma.
- Patient has severe tachycardia, fever, altered mental status, and left ventricular dysfunction.

CONGESTIVE CARDIAC FAILURE

- It occurs in about 10% cases of severe hyperthyroidism.
- Changes in the heart caused by pregnancy together with effect of hyperthyroidism on heart are responsible for it.
- PET, anemia, hemorrhage predispose to CCF[7]

OBSTETRICAL COMPLICATIONS

Maternal Complications

- Miscarriage
- PET (risk increased by fivefolds)
- Preterm delivery (risk increased by 10-folds)
- Placental abruption
- Venous thromboembolism

Fetal Complications

- Fetal growth restriction (FGR)
- Prematurity

- Intrauterine fetal demise (IUFD)
- Fetal goiter
- Hyperthyroidism
- Hypothyroidism
- Congenital anomalies[8]
- Fetal complications are due to direct toxic effect of T4/T3, thyrotropin receptor antibodies (TRaB) induced hyperthyroidism,[9] antithyroid drugs which can cause fetal anomalies (methimazole) or hypothyroidism
- Fetal thyroid gland reaches maturity by 20 weeks of gestation. Now, it can respond to antithyroid drugs as well as to TRAb. Hence, fetus can have hypo- or hyperthyroidism.
- Large fetal goiter will extend the neck and result in dystocia/lower segment cesarean section (LSCS)
- Goiter may compress trachea and esophagus which can lead to asphyxia or polyhydramnios, respectively. Polyhydramnios is responsible for preterm labor.
- Ultrasonography is helpful in differentiating between fetal hypothyroidism and hyperthyroidism **(Table 2)**.[10]

Fetal anomalies are caused by antithyroid drugs particularly if exposure occurs between 6 and 10 weeks of gestation.

Methimazole-induced defects are observed in 2–4% babies.

Typically, there can be aplasia cutis, choanal atresia, esophageal atresia, facial abnormalities, omphalocele.

PTU and MMZ can cause fetal anomalies but that caused by PTU has less severity.

TABLE 2: Sonographic differences between fetal hypothyroidism and hyperthyroidism.

USG feature		***Points***
FHR	Tachycardia	1
	Normal	0
Goiter vascularization	Central	1
	Peripheral or absent	0
Fetal movements	Normal	1
	increased	0
Bone maturation	Accelerated	-1
	Normal	0
	Delayed	1

Score > 2 suggests "Hyperthyroidism"
Score < 2 suggests "Hypothyroidism"

MANAGEMENT OF HYPERTHYROIDISM IN PREGNANCY

- Most of the patients can be managed by medical therapy. Only a few selected may need surgical treatment as well.
- Obviously, the mainstay of treatment is antithyroid drugs (ATD). There may be a need to add β-blockers in some patients.
- Methimazole/Carbimazole (MMZ) and propylthiouracil (PTU) are used in pregnancy.
- Radioactive iodine is contraindicated.
- MMZ and PTU act by inhibiting synthesis of thyroid hormones. They also have immunosuppressive activity. In addition to that PTU prevents peripheral conversion of T4–T3.
- Methimazole is converted to carbimazole which is biologically active.
- MMZ are long-acting drugs so that they are administered once or twice a day.
- PTU has to be consumed thrice a day.
- Dose MMZ 10–20 mg once or twice a day.
- PTU 50–100 mg thrice a day.

GOALS OF TREATMENT

Adequate control of maternal hyperthyroidism so as to prevent its complications in mother, fetus, and neonate:

- The fetus/neonate should neither develop hypothyroidism nor hyperthyroidism.
- T4 levels must be kept at just below the upper range of normal value so as to avoid fetal hypothyroidism as fetal thyroid gland is highly sensitive to ATD.
- TSH levels are less important than T4 levels.
- Contrary to common belief, both MMZ and PTU have potential to cause fetal anomalies.
- But, PTU is a lesser evil as anomalies due to it are less severe.[11]
- In view of that it is recommended by the American Thyroid Association (ATS) to administer PTU in 1st trimester of pregnancy and up to 16 weeks.
- The patient already on MMZ contemplating pregnancy should switch over to PTU.
- Long-term use of PTU is associated with hepatotoxicity. Therefore, beyond 16 weeks, MMZ should be administered.[12]
- PTU induced hepatotoxicity occurs at median duration of 120 days.
- Dosage ratio of 1:20 is advised while switching over from one drug to other, e.g., MMZ 15 mg/day = 300 mg PTU (in three divided doses per day).
- During the course of treatment, pregnant lady is monitored with following investigations:

- T4 and T3 levels with TSH every 2–6 weeks T4 responds but T3 may remain high. TSH remains suppressed for several months.
- Thyrotropin-receptor antibodies at diagnosis, 18–22 weeks and at 32–34 weeks

High titer of antibodies in 3rd trimester predicts neonatal hyperthyroidism

- Liver function tests every 4 weeks: If SGPT/SGOT levels are thrice the normal values, PTU must be discontinued.
- Leukocyte count every 4 weeks (to identify agranulocytosis)
  It should be checked daily if the patient has febrile illness.

Side Effects of Antithyroid Drugs

- Overall about 13% patients on ATD develop side effects.
- Nausea/vomiting are common.
- Pruritus, rash is observed in 6% with MMZ 3% with PTU
- Cutaneous reaction may appear in 24% cases with both MMZ and PTU, 18–22 days after starting the treatment.
- Agranulocytosis occurs within 69 days after initiating the drugs in 0.2–0.7%, more common due to PTU.
- Hepatotoxicity can develop as early as 28 days indicated by rise in SGPT levels.
- It is in the form of hepatocellular necrosis in 2.7% PTU users. While MMZ causes cholestasis in 0.4%.

INDICATIONS FOR SURGICAL TREATMENT

The ideal time for surgical treatment is before pregnancy. However, it can be done in 2nd trimester of pregnancy. It is indicated in following conditions:

- Adverse effects of ATD
- The need of very high doses of drugs
- Noncompliant patient
- Large goiter compressing trachea

PRECONCEPTION COUNSELING

- The best possible outcome of pregnancy is ensured if the woman enters pregnancy with well-controlled hyperthyroidism.
- The would-be parents should be explained the mutual effects of pregnancy and thyroid dysfunction on each other.
- They must know the need of switching over of ATDs in different trimesters of pregnancy.
- The occasional undesired effects of TRAb and ATDs on fetus/neonate needs discussion.
- The woman embarking on pregnancy has to undergo frequent investigations for good control of hyperthyroidism.

- If required, radioactive iodine or surgery is to be used to control hyperthyroidism before pregnancy.

CONCLUSION

Hyperthyroidism in pregnancy, though less common than hypothyroidism, poses significant risks to the mother, fetus, and neonate if unrecognized or inadequately treated. Physiological changes of pregnancy alter thyroid function tests, often masking or mimicking disease, making accurate diagnosis dependent on a clear understanding of trimester-specific reference ranges and appropriate laboratory interpretation. Differentiating pathological hyperthyroidism—particularly Graves' disease—from transient gestational thyrotoxicosis is crucial, as management strategies and prognostic implications differ substantially.

Timely diagnosis, careful classification, and judicious use of antithyroid drugs remain the cornerstone of management. The primary therapeutic goal is to maintain maternal euthyroidism while avoiding fetal hypo- or hyperthyroidism, necessitating close biochemical and clinical monitoring throughout pregnancy. Awareness of potential maternal, obstetric, and fetal complications, along with early identification of high-risk cases, can significantly reduce morbidity and mortality.

Preconception counseling and multidisciplinary care involving obstetricians, endocrinologists, and pediatricians play a pivotal role in optimizing outcomes. With appropriate planning, regular surveillance, and individualized treatment, most women with hyperthyroidism can expect a successful pregnancy and favorable maternal and neonatal outcomes.

REFERENCES

1. Soldin OP, Tractenberg RE, Hollowell JG, Jonklaas J, Janicic N, Soldin SJ. Trimester specific changes in maternal thyroid hormone, thyrotropin, and thyroglobulin concentration during gestation: trends and associations across trimesters in iodine sufficiency. Thyroid. 2004;14:1084-90.
2. Goodwin TM, Montoro M, Mestman JH. Transient hyperthyroidism and hyperemesis gravidarum: clinical aspects. Am J Obstet Gynecol. 1992;167:648-52.
3. Goldman AM, Mestman JH. Transient nonautoimmune hyperthyroidism of early pregnancy. J Thyroid Res. 2011;2011:142413.
4. Yoshihara A, Noh JY, Mukasa K, Suzuki M, Ohye H, Matsumoto M, et al. Serum human chorionic gonadotropin levels and thyroid hormone levels in gestational transient thyrotoxicosis: Is the serum hCG level useful for differentiating between active Graves' disease and GTT? Endocr J. 2015;62:557-60.
5. Verberg MF, Gillott DJ, Al-Fardan N, Grudzinskas JG. Hyperemesis gravidarum, a literature review. Hum Reprod Update. 2005;11:527-39.
6. Tina Ngan, Tin Yan, et al. Maternal and obstetric outcomes among women with thyroid storm in pregnancy: a population-based study of 4.2 million births. American Journal of Obstetrics & Gynecology, Volume 216, Issue 1, S460 - S461.

7. Sheffield JS, Cunningham FG. Thyrotoxicosis and heart failure that complicate pregnancy. Am J Ostet Gynecol. 2004;190:211-7.
8. Patil-Sisodia K, Mestman JH. Graves' hyperthyroidism and pregnancy: a clinical update. Endocr Pract. 2010;16:118-21.
9. Polak M, Le Gac I, Vuillard E, Guibourdenche J, Leger J, Toubert ME, et al. Fetal and neonatal thyroid function in relation to maternal Graves' disease. Best Pract Res Clin Endocrinol Metab. 2004;18:289-302.
10. Huel C, Guibourdenche J, Vuillard E, Ouahba J, Piketty M, Oury JF, et al. Use of ultrasound to distinguish between fetal hyperthyroidism and hypothyroidism on discovery of a goiter. Ultrasound Obstet Gynecol. 2009;33:412-20.
11. Andersen SL, Lönn S, Vestergaard P, Törring O. Birth defects after use of antithyroid drugs in early pregnancy: a Swedish nationwide study. Eur J Endocrinol. 2017;177(4):369-78.
12. Ross DS, Burch HB, Cooper DS, Greenlee MC, Laurberg P, Maia AL, et al. 2016 American Thyroid Association Guidelines for Diagnosis and Management of Hyperthyroidism and Other Causes of Thyrotoxicosis. Thyroid. 2016;26(10):1343-421.

CHAPTER 4

Hypothyroidism in Pregnancy

Vaishali Korde-Nayak, Aishwarya Agrawal

INTRODUCTION

The thyroid gland plays a pivotal role in metabolic regulation through its hormones triiodothyronine (T_3) and thyroxine (T_4). These are essential not only for metabolic homeostasis but also for somatic growth and, most critically, for normal brain development. Their synthesis is governed by the hypothalamic–pituitary–thyroid axis, ensuring physiologic balance across organ systems. Even minor disturbances in thyroid function can meaningfully influence reproductive physiology and are now recognized as important contributors to subfertility and adverse pregnancy outcomes.[1]

Thyroid dysfunction is the most common endocrine disorder among women of reproductive age.[1] Hypothyroidism is defined biochemically by elevated thyroid-stimulating hormone (TSH), with further classification guided by free T_4 concentrations: overt hypothyroidism is characterized by low free T_4, whereas subclinical hypothyroidism features normal free T_4 despite a raised TSH.[2] Symptomatic individuals with presence of high levels of antithyroid peroxidase or antithyroglobulin antibodies are also included in this spectrum of subclinical thyroid disease.[2,3]

Current epidemiological estimates indicate that 2–4% of pregnant women have subclinical hypothyroidism, while 0.3–1% of reproductive-age women manifest overt disease.[3] According to the FOGSI 2022 report, the global prevalence ranges from 1.5 to 4%, whereas the Indian prevalence is significantly higher at 11%.[4] Worldwide, iodine deficiency remains the leading etiology of hypothyroidism.[5]

A review by Amanda Jeffreys et al., published in *The Obstetrician and Gynaecologist* (Royal College of Obstetricians and Gynaecologists), provides a detailed enumeration of the recognized causes of hypothyroidism, offering a comprehensive framework for understanding its etiopathogenesis.[1]

CAUSES

Causes of hypothyroidism are given in **Table 1**

PHYSIOLOGY

The physiology of the maternal–fetal thyroid axis is highly interdependent. In the mother, thyrotropin-releasing hormone (TRH) stimulates pituitary secretion of TSH, thereby augmenting the synthesis of T_3 and T_4. Due to the increased requirement of thyroid hormones in pregnancy, thyroid gland

TABLE 1: Causes of hypothyroidism[1]

Category	*Subtype*	*Causes*
Primary hypothyroidism	Autoimmune	• Hashimoto's thyroiditis • Atrophic thyroiditis
	Iatrogenic	• Radioactive iodine therapy • Thyroidectomy • Antithyroid drugs
	Transient	• Subacute (De Quervain's) thyroiditis • Postpartum thyroiditis
	Iodine deficiency	• Dietary or environmental iodine deficiency
Secondary hypothyroidism	—	• Pituitary failure • Pituitary tumor
Tertiary hypothyroidism	—	• Hypothalamic failure

enlarges marginally, typically insufficient to produce clinically appreciable thyromegaly. In early pregnancy, rising estrogen concentrations leads to a marked elevation in thyroid-binding globulin (TBG), resulting in increased circulating total T_3 and T_4 levels. However, free T_3 and free T_4 concentrations remain unaffected, making them the preferred biochemical parameters of choice for diagnosing thyroid dysfunction in pregnancy. The fetal thyroid gland becomes functional only after approximately 12 weeks of gestation, gradually increasing endogenous hormone production thereafter. TSH does not cross the placenta, and thus exerts no direct fetal effects. Consequently, the fetus relies heavily on transplacental transfer of maternal thyroxine, a dependence that persists throughout gestation. Even at term, nearly one-third of fetal thyroid hormone content is maternally derived.[4] Maternal thyroxine plays an indispensable role in fetal neurodevelopment. Any alteration in its levels is negatively associated with reduced cortical brain volume and may have long-term neurocognitive consequences.

THYROID AUTOIMMUNITY

Autoimmune thyroid disease is characterized by the presence of thyroid-specific autoantibodies, most commonly antibodies directed against thyroglobulin, the substrate required for thyroid hormone synthesis and storage, and antithyroid peroxidase (anti-TPO) antibodies, enzyme involved in thyroid hormone synthesis. Their presence triggers an autoimmune reaction leading to progressive lymphocytic infiltration of the thyroid gland, followed by fibrosis and architectural distortion. This has a negative influence on fertility and pregnancy outcomes.[5] Approximately 5–10% of women harboring thyroid autoantibodies develop hypothyroidism during pregnancy.[1] These women have a 3–5-fold increase in early pregnancy loss, a threefold higher risk of placental abruption, and a 1.5-fold elevation in the likelihood of preterm birth.[3] However, as per the American College of Obstetricians and Gynecologists (ACOG), there is no recommendation for universal screening of these antibodies in pregnancy.[6]

MATERNAL AND FETAL EFFECTS

It is now well-established that both overt and subclinical hypothyroidism during pregnancy contribute to a wide spectrum of maternal and fetal complications, culminating in significant adverse obstetric outcomes. In women of reproductive age, it is associated with increased rates of infertility and recurrent early pregnancy loss. Antenatal complications include higher risk of maternal anemia, preeclampsia, cardiac dysfunction, placental abruption, and postpartum hemorrhage. Consequently, fetal and neonatal outcomes are disproportionately affected, which include congenital malformations, prematurity, low-birth weight, stillbirth, neonatal respiratory distress, and increased need for neonatal intensive care unit (NICU) admission. Congenital hypothyroidism can be seen in cases of autoimmune hypothyroidism. Such neonates may also have neurodevelomental delays.[1,3,6-8]

MANAGEMENT

Antenatal Management

Given the substantial maternal–fetal risks associated with inadequately treated hypothyroidism, optimization of thyroid status prior to conception is ideal. Levothyroxine, the synthetic form of thyroxine, remains the treatment of choice, with a prepregnancy TSH target of <2.5 mIU/L for women planning conception.

Guideline positions on screening vary. The American Thyroid Association (ATA), European Thyroid Association (ETA), and the Royal College of Obstetricians and Gynecologists (RCOG) acknowledge insufficient evidence to support universal thyroid screening in pregnancy, while the American College of Obstetricians and Gynecologists (ACOG) recommends against universal screening. In contrast, the 2019 joint guideline by the Indian Thyroid Society (ITS) and FOGSI advocates universal screening for all pregnant women.

Initial evaluation consists of serum TSH, which identifies primary hypothyroidism, and free T_4, which differentiates overt from subclinical disease. Testing should be performed at the first antenatal visit. Thyroid antibody testing may be considered in high-risk women—those with recurrent pregnancy loss, prior preterm birth, goiter, history of thyroid surgery, body mass index (BMI) > 30 kg/m^2, family history of thyroid disease, or coexisting autoimmune disorders.[1-8]

Physiological changes in pregnancy increase maternal levothyroxine requirements as early as 5 weeks, with stabilization by 20 weeks. Women with pre-existing overt hypothyroidism should have TSH assessed immediately upon confirmation of pregnancy, and their dose increased by ~25 µg/day or ~30% of the prepregnancy dose.

For newly diagnosed overt hypothyroidism, levothyroxine is initiated at 1.6–2.0 µg/kg/day. TSH targets are trimester-specific: 0.1–2.5 mIU/L (first trimester), 0.2–3.0 mIU/L (second trimester), and 0.3–3.0 mIU/L (third trimester). Monitoring is performed every 4–6 weeks until mid-gestation, and once again around 28 weeks, with dose titration as needed.

In antibody-positive women with TSH 4–10 mIU/L, or in those with TSH > 10 mIU/L with normal free T_4, levothyroxine 50–100 µg/day is recommended. Women with autoimmune thyroid disease require TSH monitoring every 4 weeks, and at least once more between 26 and 32 weeks, due to their increased risk of decompensation.[4-8]

Postnatal Management

Following delivery, thyroid physiology generally returns to baseline. Women with pre-existing hypothyroidism should revert to their prepregnancy levothyroxine dose, with TSH reassessed at 6 weeks postpartum.

Flowchart 1: FOGSI guidelines on management of hypothyroidism in pregnancy.[4]

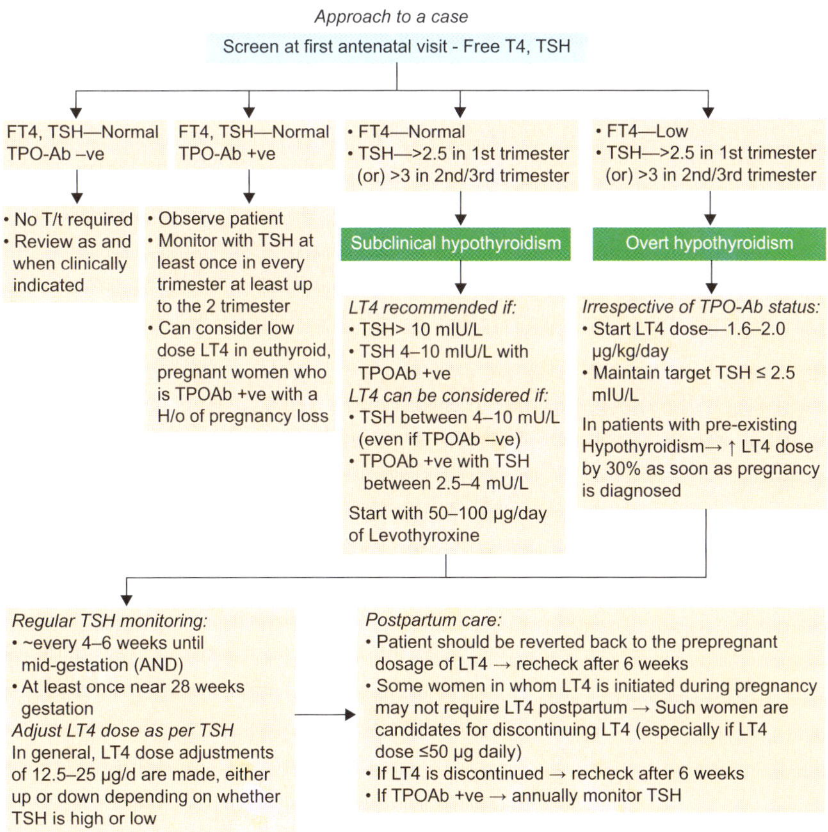

For women diagnosed with overt hypothyroidism for the first time during pregnancy, levothyroxine may be discontinued postpartum, followed by repeat TSH testing at 6 weeks to determine the need for continued therapy.

If anti-TPO antibodies are positive, long-term surveillance is essential, and annual TSH testing is recommended due to the heightened risk of developing permanent hypothyroidism.[4]

CONCLUSION

Thyroid disease in pregnancy can have significant adverse effects from conception to delivery and even in postpartum period both on the mother and the baby. Anemia is prevalent among pregnant population in our county and it is also a complication seen in hypothyroidism. However, with universal screening in all antenatal patients, timely diagnosis and appropriate treatment can help to invert future complications ensuring good maternal and fetal outcome. This can also be achieved with prepregnancy optimization of thyroid status in cases of overt hypothyroidism **(Flowchart 1)**.

REFERENCES

1. Jefferys A, Vanderpump M, Yasmin E. Thyroid dysfunction and reproductive health. Obstet Gynaecol. 2015;17(1):39-45.
2. Yadav V, Dabar D, Goel AD, Bairwa M, Sood A, Prasad P, et al. Prevalence of Hypothyroidism in Pregnant Women in India: A Meta-Analysis of Observational Studies. J Thyroid Res. 2021;2021(1):5515831.
3. Cunningham FG, Leveno KJ, Dashe JS, Hoffman BL, Spong CY, Casey BM. Endocrine abnormalities. Maternal and surgical complications. In: Cunningham FG., Lenovo KJ, Dashe JS, Hoffman BL, Spong CY, Casey BM (Eds). Williams Obstetrics, 26th edition. United States: McGraw Hill; 2022.
4. Federation of Obstetric and Gynecological Societies of India. Hypothyroidism in pregnancy. Mumbai: Federation of Obstetric and Gynecological Societies of India; 2022.
5. Dhillon-Smith RK, Boelaert K, Jeve YB, Maheshwari A, Coomarasamy A; on behalf of Royal College of Obstetricians and Gynaecologists. Subclinical hypothyroidism and antithyroid autoantibodies in women with subfertility or recurrent pregnancy loss. Scientific Impact Paper no. 78. BJOG. 2022;129:e75-e88.
6. Kilpatrick SJ. ACOG Guidelines at a Glance Thyroid Disease in Pregnancy. Obstet Gynecol. 2015.
7. Teng W, Shan Z, Patil-Sisodia K, Cooper DS. Hypothyroidism in pregnancy. Lancet Diabetes Endocrinol. 2013;1(3):228-37.
8. Indian Thyroid Society and Federation of Obstetric and Gynecological Societies of India. Recommendations for the management of Thyroid Dysfunction in Pregnancy. Guidelines by Indian Thyroid Society and Federation of Obstetric and Gynecological Societies of India. 2019.

CHAPTER 5

Postpartum Thyroiditis

Uma Wankhede

INTRODUCTION

Postpartum thyroiditis (PPT) is the occurrence of any type of thyroid disease other than Graves' disease during the 1st year after delivery in women who never had any thyroid disorder in their life. An inflammatory autoimmune process is the cause of this condition. In the classic form of PPT, initially there is thyrotoxicosis with increased thyroid function which is followed by transient hypothyroidism where the thyroid function declines followed by return to the euthyroid state by the end of the 1st year after delivery.

In the different clinical presentations of PPT, approximately 25% of patients present with the classical form, 25% presenting with only thyrotoxicosis, and 50% presenting with isolated hypothyroidism.[1]

CLINICAL FEATURES OF POSTPARTUM THYROIDITIS

Thyrotoxic Phase

The thyrotoxic phase of PPT typically occurs first between 2nd and 6th month of delivery with some patients reporting thyrotoxic symptoms as late as up to 1 year postpartum. All episodes of thyrotoxicosis resolve spontaneously without any treatment.

Hypothyroid Phase

The hypothyroid phase of PPT occurs from 3 to 12 months postpartum but about 10–20% of patients remain in permanent hypothyroidism and fail to revert to euthyroid state.[2]

PATHOPHYSIOLOGY AND AUTOIMMUNE BASIS

Postpartum thyroiditis is an autoimmune disorder characterized by the presence of thyroid autoantibodies (TPO-Ab and T gAb),lymphocyte abnormalities, complement activation, increased levels of immunoglobulin G (IgG)-1, increased natural killer (NK) cell activity, and specific human leukocyte antigen (HLA) haplotypes. This derangement in immune function may not cause any problems in pregnancy.[3]

Those women who have thyroid autoantibodies in pregnancy are at high risk of developing PPT after their delivery ranging from 33 to 50% risk. The higher the antibody titer, the greater the risk of developing PPT. The occurrence of PPT in the postpartum period reflects the rebound of the immune system in the postpartum period after the relative immune suppression caused by pregnancy.

DIFFERENTIAL DIAGNOSIS: POSTPARTUM THYROIDITIS VERSUS GRAVES' DISEASE

The main problem is the differentiation of thyrotoxicosis due to PPT from Graves' disease. This is critically important as both conditions have completely different clinical course and completely different management. The timing of onset may provide some clue about etiology. Mostly patients who develop thyrotoxicosis within the first 3 months after delivery have PPT while patients who develop thyrotoxicosis late after delivery, after 6 months or later may be having Graves' disease. So, early onset of thyrotoxicosis is more likely to be PPT than Graves' disease.

Thyroid-stimulating hormone receptors are positive in Graves' disease in nearly all cases and are typically negative in PPT although some mixed type diseases are seen. An elevated T4:T3 suggests the presence of PPT. Physical stigmata of Graves' disease like exophthalmos or goiter with bruit, if present, are diagnostic. The radioactive iodine uptake is elevated or normal in Graves' disease and low in the thyrotoxic phase of postpartum thyroiditis (PPD), but it is better to avoid radioactive diagnostic procedure in lactating patients. Due to shorter half-life I-231 or technetium scans (Tc-99m) may be used in women who are breastfeeding if breast milk is pumped and discarded for several days after the scan has been performed.

EPIDEMIOLOGY AND RISK FACTORS

The prevalence of PPT is approximately 5% of all deliveries. Women with other autoimmune disorders have an increased risk of PPT due to presence of associated antibodies. The prevalence of PPT is 3–4 times higher in women with type 1 diabetes mellitus as compared to nondiabetic women. The frequency of PPT is 25% in chronic viral hepatitis, 14% in women with SLE, 44% in women with previous history of Graves' disease, and 27% in patients with antipituitary antibodies. Women who recover from PPT have a 70% risk of developing PPT in subsequent pregnancy. Women on thyroxine therapy due to Hashimotos thyroiditis may develop PPT if their thyroid gland is not completely atrophic. So, one must be watchful for PPT in postpartum mothers who have associated other autoimmune diseases or who have a past history of PPT in previous pregnancy.[4]

SYMPTOMS AND CLINICAL PRESENTATION

Postpartum thyroiditis is a painless condition and most women are asymptomatic or mildly symptomatic in the thyrotoxic phase. This is because the degree of increase in thyroid hormones is generally less, and T4 levels are more increased than T3 levels. Some patients can be present in the 1st year postpartum with vague symptoms like irritability, heat intolerance, fatigue and palpitations. In many cases, the diagnosis can only be made if the condition is thought of.

The hypothyroid phase of PPT is generally more symptomatic. Symptoms in the hypothyroid phase of PPT may include cold intolerance, dry skin, fatigue, impaired concentration, and paresthesia. Patients of PPT who are TPO antibodies present are generally more symptomatic than patients who are TPO antibodies negative.

Many studies have shown a relationship between thyroid antibodies and postpartum depression, while other studies show no association between the presence of microsomal antibodies and postpartum depression.

All patients of depression including postpartum depression must be evaluated for thyroid dysfunction along with other tests.

MANAGEMENT OF POSTPARTUM THYROIDITIS

Treatment of the thyrotoxic phase depend on the symptoms present. ATDs (PTU and MMI) are ineffective in treating the thyrotoxic phase of the disease because it is a destructive type of thyroiditis in which thyroid hormone synthesis is not increased. Symptoms are usually mild. In rare cases where symptoms are clinically significant, propranolol at the lowest possible dose to alleviate symptoms may be used. Therapy is typically required for a few weeks only. ATDs are not required for the thyrotoxic phase of PPT.

After the resolution of the thyrotoxic phase of PPT, serum TSH should be measured after 4–8 weeks to screen for hypothyroidism.[5]

In women with significant symptoms of hypothyroidism, those currently lactating or those women who are actively attempting pregnancy treatment should be started. LT4 should be started in all patients who are symptomatic, lactating or attempting pregnancy if the TSH is raised. If treatment is delayed, thyroid function should be reassessed every 4–8 weeks until euthyroidism is established and women should be counseled to use contraception.

The length of time that LT4 should be used is not definite. Guiding principles are to maintain a euthyroid state in women who are symptomatic, lactating or trying to achieve pregnancy. The lowest possible dose of LT4 to maintain patient euthyroid should be given. Tapering LT4 doses in order to determine whether the hypothyroid phase of PPT was transitory or permanent can begin by 12 months postpartum. Tapering should be gradual and serum TSH levels should be checked every 6–8 weeks.

Tapering of LT4 should be avoided if women is symptomatic, lactating or actively attempting pregnancy.

LONG-TERM OUTCOMES

The impact of PPT on long-term thyroid function has been evaluated in several studies. Almost 50% of women in whom the hypothyroid phase of PPT initially resolves will ultimately go on to develop permanent hypothyroidism. Factors associated with increased risk of developing permanent hypothyroidism include multiparity, thyroid hypoechogenicity on ultrasound, greater severity of the initial hypothyroidism, higher TPOAb titers, increased maternal age, and history of pregnancy losses.

Women with a past history of PPT should have their TSH levels checked annually to evaluate for the development of permanent hypothyroidism.[6]

Ther is no role of iodine or LT4 during pregnancy in women who are antibody positive to help in prevention of PPT in them. Only one must be watchful for the possible onset of PPT and manage it correctly and on time.

CONCLUSION

Postpartum thyroiditis is a common autoimmune thyroid disorder occurring within the 1st year after delivery in women who were euthyroid prior to pregnancy. Its clinical presentation is variable, ranging from transient thyrotoxicosis followed by hypothyroidism to isolated thyrotoxic or hypothyroid phases. Although the thyrotoxic phase is typically mild and self-limiting, the hypothyroid phase is more frequently symptomatic and may progress to permanent hypothyroidism in a significant proportion of women.

Early recognition of PPT is essential, particularly to differentiate it from Graves' disease, as the management and prognosis of these conditions differ markedly. The presence of thyroid autoantibodies, characteristic biochemical patterns, timing of symptom onset, and clinical features aid in accurate diagnosis. Given the association of PPT with other autoimmune disorders and its high recurrence rate in subsequent pregnancies, women at risk require close postpartum surveillance.

Management is largely supportive, with β-blockers reserved for symptomatic thyrotoxicosis and levothyroxine therapy indicated during the hypothyroid phase in symptomatic women, those who are breastfeeding, or those planning future pregnancies. Long-term follow-up is crucial, as a substantial proportion of affected women ultimately develop permanent hypothyroidism. Routine screening for thyroid dysfunction, especially in women with postpartum depression or prior PPT, is therefore warranted. A structured approach to diagnosis, treatment, and follow-up can ensure optimal maternal health and prevent long-term thyroid morbidity.

REFERENCES

1. Lazarus JH. Reduction of post-partum thyroiditis. Eur J Endocrinol. 1998;139:12-3.

2. Rot E, Uberti E. Post-partum thyroiditis - a clinical update. Eur J Endocrinol. 2002;146:275-9.
3. Harris B, Othman S, Davies JA, Weppner GJ, Richards CJ, Newcombe RG, et al. Association between postpartum thyroid dysfunction and thyroid antibodies and depression. BMJ. 1992;305(6846):152-6.
4. Othman S, Phillips DI, Parkes AB, Richards CJ, Harris B, Fung H, et al. A long-term follow-up of postpartum thyroiditis. Clin Endocrinol. 1990;32:559-64.
5. Stagnaro-Green A. Approach to the patient with post-partum thyroiditis. J Clin Endocrinol Metab. 2012;97(2):334-42.
6. Samuels MH. Subacute, silent and postpartum thyroiditis. Med Clin North Am. 2012;96(2):223-33.

CHAPTER 6

Thyroid Screening in Pregnancy: Whom, When, and How?

Shweta Avinash Khade, Smurti Kamble

INTRODUCTION

Pregnancy induces substantial physiological alterations in thyroid function, rendering both clinical assessment and interpretation of thyroid function tests more complex.[1] These adaptive changes are essential to meet increased maternal and fetal metabolic demands, particularly during early gestation. Thyroid dysfunction during pregnancy has been consistently linked with adverse maternal and neonatal outcomes; however, timely diagnosis and appropriate treatment can effectively mitigate these risks.

Globally, thyroid disorders complicate approximately 5–11% of pregnancies. Indian data, supported by studies and consensus statements from the Federation of Obstetric and Gynecological Societies of India (FOGSI) and the Indian Thyroid Association (ITA), indicate a considerably higher prevalence, often ranging between 10 and 30%.[2] Although hyperthyroidism affects a smaller proportion of pregnant women (approximately 0.1–0.4%), it is associated with disproportionately higher maternal and fetal morbidity.[3]

Current recommendations on thyroid screening in pregnancy vary among professional bodies, including the American Thyroid Association (ATA), American College of Obstetricians and Gynecologists (ACOG), Endocrine Society, European Thyroid Association (ETA), FOGSI, and ITA, particularly with respect to universal versus targeted screening strategies.

WHOM, WHEN, AND HOW TO SCREEN?

Whom to Screen?

- *Universal screening:* FOGSI and the Indian Thyroid Association recommend thyroid screening for all pregnant women during early 1st trimester.[4,5]
- *High-risk women (as per selective screening guidelines):* History of thyroid disease or goiter, autoimmune disorders including type 1 diabetes mellitus, prior head or neck irradiation, recurrent pregnancy loss or infertility, and clinical features suggestive of thyroid dysfunction.
- *Symptomatic women:* Any pregnant woman exhibiting signs or symptoms of hypo- or hyperthyroidism.

When to Screen?

- *Preconception:* Ideally for women planning pregnancy.

- *Early pregnancy:* Best done early (ideally before 9 weeks or at first prenatal booking). Maternal thyroid hormones are critical for fetal neurodevelopment during the 1st trimester, as the fetal thyroid gland remains functionally inactive until approximately 18–20 weeks of gestation.
- *Follow-up testing:* If abnormal results are detected, thyroid function should be reassessed every 4–6 weeks until mid-pregnancy, with at least one repeat assessment around 30 weeks of gestation.

How to Screen and Monitor?

- *Primary investigation:* Serum thyroid-stimulating hormone (TSH).
- *Additional investigations:* If TSH levels are abnormal, free T4 (fT4) and thyroid peroxidase antibodies (TPOAb) should be tested to determine the type and cause of the dysfunction.
- *Reference ranges:* Interpretation should be based on trimester-specific reference ranges whenever available.

UNIVERSAL VERSUS SELECTIVE SCREENING

The principal controversy in antenatal thyroid care revolves around universal screening of all pregnant women versus selective screening of those considered high-risk.

Selective Screening (Recommended by ATA, ACOG, and RCOG)

Most current major guidelines recommend screening only women with specific risk factors for thyroid disease.[6-8] Risk factors include:

- History of thyroid dysfunction or goiter
- Symptoms suggestive of thyroid dysfunction
- Presence of thyroid antibodies (TPOAbs) in the serum
- History of preterm delivery or miscarriage
- Type 1 diabetes mellitus or other autoimmune disorders
- History of head or neck irradiation
- Age >30 years
- Family history of thyroid disease
- Morbid obesity

Universal Screening (FOGSI and ITA)

FOGSI and ITA advocate universal screening, citing evidence that targeted approaches may fail to identify up to 30–55% of women with thyroid dysfunction, including cases of overt hypothyroidism.

- Thyroid dysfunction can have severe consequences on pregnancy outcomes, including preeclampsia, miscarriage, fetal death in the uterus, premature birth, and low-birth weight. Children can present with lower IQ and learning difficulties due to the deleterious impact on the neurocognitive development of the fetus.[4] Correct and timely diagnoses are essential to offer appropriate treatment to pregnant women to prevent complications.

- The goal of universal screening of maternal TSH levels is the diagnosis of dysfunction at the prenatal or early gestational stage so that therapeutic intervention can be performed before crucial irreversible changes in fetal development occur.
- Identifying and treating thyroid dysfunction can improve neonatal and maternal outcomes. Moreover, the cost of treatment is reasonable. Given the high prevalence of thyroid disorders in India and the relative affordability of treatment, universal screening is considered a cost-effective public health strategy.
- While universal screening identifies more cases, randomized controlled trials evaluating treatment of subclinical hypothyroidism have yielded inconsistent evidence regarding improvement in maternal and fetal outcomes, leading several international societies to continue endorsing selective screening.
- FOGSI and ITA strongly recommend universal thyroid screening in early pregnancy (1st trimester), ideally at the first prenatal visit, using trimester-specific TSH thresholds (e.g., <2.5 mIU/L in the 1st trimester) to prevent adverse outcomes such as preterm birth and fetal complications.

FIRST TRIMESTER THYROID-STIMULATING HORMONE TARGETS AND REFERENCE RANGES

Pregnancy alters thyroid physiology, so trimester-specific TSH reference ranges are crucial for accurate diagnosis **(Table 1)**.[4]

TABLE 1: Trimester-specific recommended thyroid-stimulating hormone (TSH) reference ranges according to international guidelines.

Guidelines	*Country*	*Trimester-specific recommended TSH reference range*
ITA guidelines 2012	India	• 1st: 2.5 mIU/L • 2nd: 3.0 mIU/L • 3rd: 3.0 mIU/L
ETA guidelines 2014	Europe	• 1st: 2.5 mIU/L • 2nd: 3.0 mIU/L • 3rd: 3.0 mIU/L
ATA guidelines 2017	America	Use locally derived reference ranges from a specified pregnant population. If the above is not available use an upper TSH reference limit of 4.0 mIU/L

TABLE 2: Types of thyroid disorders in pregnancy and the postpartum period.

Type of disorder	*Description*	*Common cause*
1. Overt hypothyroidism	The thyroid is severely underactive, with high TSH and low free T4 levels	Hashimoto's thyroiditis (autoimmune) or iodine deficiency worldwide
2. Subclinical hypothyroidism	A milder form where TSH levels are high, but free T4 levels remain within the normal range for pregnancy	Hashimoto's thyroiditis is the most common cause in iodine-sufficient areas
3. Overt hyperthyroidism	The thyroid is overactive, producing excess hormones, with low TSH and high free T4 levels	*Graves' disease* (an autoimmune disease) accounts for most cases
4 Subclinical hyperthyroidism	A mild form in which TSH is low, but free T4 is normal for the gestational age	This is often due to high hCG levels in early pregnancy (gestational transient thyrotoxicosis)
5. Postpartum thyroiditis	Thyroid inflammation within 1 year after delivery, often involving a transient hyperthyroid phase followed by a hypothyroid phase	Autoimmune conditions are more common in women with pre-existing thyroid antibodies
6. Gestational transient thyrotoxicosis (GTT)	Temporary hyperthyroidism in the 1st trimester is caused by high levels of human chorionic gonadotropin (hCG), which usually resolves spontaneously	High hCG levels are often associated with severe morning sickness (hyperemesis gravidarum)

Thyroid disorders during pregnancy can be broadly categorized into conditions of underactivity (hypothyroidism) and overactivity (hyperthyroidism), which can be overt or subclinical.[9] Postpartum thyroiditis is another common condition that occurs after delivery.

There are six key types of thyroid disorders that can affect women during or after pregnancy **(Table 2)**.

Early diagnosis and treatment are crucial for managing these conditions to ensure the health of both mothers and babies. Women with a history of thyroid issues or a family history of autoimmune disorders are at a higher risk and should be closely monitored by their healthcare providers.

WHEN TO REPEAT TESTING (MONITORING)?

Monitoring is essential throughout pregnancy, especially for women undergoing treatment or those with thyroid antibodies.

- *Frequency:* TSH (with fT4 when indicated) should be assessed every 4–6 weeks until 20 weeks of gestation, and once again in the 3rd trimester.

TABLE 3: Algorithm for evaluation and management of thyroid dysfunction in pregnancy.

Step	*Test*	*Result*	*Next action/Diagnosis*
1	Initial screening (First antenatal visit)	Measure thyroid-stimulating hormone (TSH) levels	Use population- or trimester-specific reference ranges. If local ranges are unavailable, the ATA recommends an upper limit of *2.5 mIU/L in the 1st trimester* and *3.0 mIU/L in the 2nd and 3rd trimesters*
2	If TSH is high	TSH > Upper limit of normal (ULN)	Measure *free T4 (FT4)*
3	Evaluate high TSH results	*TSH* > ULN and *FT4* < lower limit of normal	Diagnosis: *Overt hypothyroidism.* Initiate levothyroxine (LT4) treatment
		TSH > ULN and *FT4* levels were within the normal range.	Diagnosis: *Subclinical hypothyroidism.* Measure *TPOAb* (thyroid peroxidase antibodies)
4	Subclinical hypothyroidism follow-up	*TPOAb positive*	Treatment with LT4 is often indicated (e.g., 50 µg/day)
		TPOAb negative	Treatment is often not initiated, and close monitoring may be required
5	If TSH is low	TSH < the lower limit of normal (LLN) (e.g., <0.1 mIU/L in the 1st trimester)	Measure *FT4* and potentially total T3
6	Evaluate low TSH results	*TSH* suppressed and *FT4* elevated	Diagnosis: *Overt hyperthyroidism.* Evaluation of the causes (e.g., Graves' disease and gestational thyrotoxicosis)
		TSH suppressed and *FT4/T3* normal	Diagnosis: *Subclinical hyperthyroidism.*
7	Monitoring	For all treated cases and high-risk patients	Monitor TSH levels every 4–6 weeks throughout pregnancy to ensure they remain within the target range

- *Dose adjustment:* For women with pre-existing hypothyroidism, the levothyroxine dose typically needs to be increased by approximately 30% upon confirmation of pregnancy (e.g., adding two extra doses per week). The dose is then titrated to maintain the TSH level within the target range.
- *Postpartum:* Thyroid function should be re-evaluated 6 weeks after delivery, and most women return to their prepregnancy levels.

PRACTICAL ALGORITHMS FOR MANAGEMENT

The recommended approach, as per guidelines from bodies such as the American Thyroid Association (ATA), emphasizes the use of trimester-specific TSH reference ranges **(Table 3)**.

CONCLUSION

- *Universal versus high-risk screening:* While some organizations, such as the American College of Obstetricians and Gynecologists (ACOG), recommend only high-risk screening, the Indian Thyroid Society, FOGSI, and other studies support universal screening as a cost-effective measure.
- *Trimester-specific ranges:* Laboratory reference ranges for TSH shift during pregnancy due to hormonal changes. Using the correct local trimester-specific ranges is crucial for accurate diagnosis.
- *Treatment goal:* The primary goal of treatment is to maintain maternal TSH levels within the optimal range, typically *≤2.5 mIU/L* in the 1st trimester and *≤3.0 mIU/L* in the 2nd and 3rd trimesters.

REFERENCES

1. Ghazal K, Moal V, Gauchez AS, Caron P, Hamdi S. Screening for thyroid disease in pregnancy: Targeted or universal?. Médecine Nucléaire. 2023;47(4):169-74.
2. Kaur H, Padda MK, Narayan R, Kaur G. Evaluation of thyroid disorders in pregnancy: prevalence and its varieties. Int J Reprod Contracept Obstet Gynecol. 2025;14(11):3857-62.
3. Singh S, Haq N, Sandhu S. Thyroid Disease and Pregnancy. [Updated 2025 Jan 19]. In: StatPearls [Internet]. Treasure Island (FL): StatPearls Publishing; 2025.
4. Recommendations for the management of Thyroid Dysfunction in Pregnancy. Guidelines by Indian Thyroid Society and Federation of Obstetric and Gynecological Societies of India. 2019.
5. Rajput R, Bajaj S, Ghosh S, Kalra P, Menon AS, Pillai MG, et al. Thyroid disorders in pregnancy: Consensus statement of Indian Thyroid Society. Thyroid Res Pract. 2021;18:89-110.
6. Alexander EK, Pearce EN, Brent GA, Brown RS, Chen H, Dosiou C, et al. Guidelines of the American Thyroid Association for the Diagnosis and Management of Thyroid Disease During Pregnancy and the Postpartum. Thyroid. 2017;27(3):315-89.
7. American College of Obstetricians and Gynecologists. Practice Bulletin No. 148: thyroid disease in pregnancy. Obstet Gynecol. 2015;125:996-1005.
8. Chan SY, Marsh MS, Gilbert J, Boelaert K, Evans C, Dhillon-Smith R, et al Management of Thyroid Disorders in Pregnancy. BJOG. 2025;132:e130-61.
9. Federation of Obstetric and Gynecological Societies of India. Hypothyroidism in pregnancy. Mumbai: Federation of Obstetric and Gynecological Societies of India; 2022.

CHAPTER 7

Thyroid Disorders in Infertility and Recurrent Pregnancy Loss

Srushti S Joshi

INTRODUCTION

Infertility affects approximately one out of six people globally,[1] and among those who do conceive, 2–5% experience recurrent pregnancy losses (RPL).[2] Importantly, women with infertility or RPL exhibit a significantly higher prevalence of thyroid dysfunction—including overt and subclinical hypothyroidism, hyperthyroidism, and thyroid autoimmunity—compared with the general population.[3,4]

The biological link between thyroid homeostasis and reproductive outcomes is well established. Thyroid hormones influence every step of the reproductive process—from follicular development and ovulation to endometrial receptivity, implantation, placental function, and fetal neurodevelopment.[5] When thyroid function is impaired, these finely tuned processes become disrupted, contributing to anovulation, diminished embryo quality, failed implantation, biochemical pregnancies, early miscarriage, and adverse obstetric outcomes.[6] Thus, the need for screening such women for thyroid disorders is increasingly being recognized.

THYROID HORMONES AND REPRODUCTIVE PHYSIOLOGY

Thyroid hormones play a critical role in female reproductive physiology through its effects on the hypothalamo-pituitary-ovarian (HPO) axis. Triiodothyronine (T3) and Thyroxine (T4) play an essential role in modulating pulsatility of gonadotrophin releasing hormone (GnRH) and pituitary secretion of follicle stimulating hormone (FSH) and luteinizing hormone (LH).[7] Even mild hypothyroidism causes elevation of prolactin levels, disrupting the delicate balance of GnRH, FSH, and LH which eventually results in anovulation and luteal phase defects.[7]

At the ovarian level, thyroid receptors are present in granulosa and stromal cells. Thyroid hormones play an important role in facilitating normal folliculogenesis, steroidogenesis and oocyte maturation.[8] Thyroid function alterations are associated with impaired oocyte development, poor oocyte quality, and often even reduced ovarian reserve, especially in the setting of thyroid autoimmunity.[9]

At the endometrial level, thyroid hormones are responsible for optimal endometrial proliferation, differentiation, and development of endometrial receptivity. Early trophoblastic tissue also shows presence of thyroid receptors, underlining the importance of thyroid homeostasis during peri-implantation and placentation stages.[10] Structural homology between human chorionic gonadotropin (hCG) and thyroid-stimulating hormone (TSH) permits partial receptor crossreactivity in early gestation, reflecting the intrinsic coupling of pregnancy physiology with maternal thyroid regulation.[11] This helps to explain why implantation and early pregnancy development are sensitive to even minor fluctuations in thyroid function.

THYROID DISORDERS

Thyroid dysfunction—including overt and subclinical hypo- and hyperthyroidism, as well as thyroid autoimmunity—can impair reproductive function. Recognition of these disorders is essential in women presenting with infertility or recurrent pregnancy losses.

Overt Hypothyroidism

This is a condition with elevated serum TSH levels along with a decrease in free T4 levels. The prevalence of overt hypothyroidism is 0.2–0.5% among subfertile women.[12] Hypothyroidism-related metabolic alterations cause subfertility as a result of anovulation and luteal phase dysfunction. Further primary hypothyroidism causes an increase in levels of thyrotropin-releasing hormone (TRH) → hyperprolactinemia[13]→ suppression of pulsatile GnRH release → further aggravates anovulation. Even if conception does occur, inadequate thyroid levels in early pregnancy impair trophoblast invasion and placental formation leading to increased chances of miscarriage in 1st trimester.[14] If left untreated, the risk or miscarriages may recur in subsequent pregnancies. In assisted reproductive technology (ART) cycles, overt hypothyroidism is associated with suboptimal ovarian response, reduced mature oocyte yield, lower fertilization rates, and compromised embryo quality.[15]

Subclinical Hypothyroidism

Conventionally subclinical hypothyroidism refers to the condition where serum TSH is elevated modestly (between 4.5 and 10 mIU/L) with free T4 levels are within normal range.[16] Often for women considering ART procedures lower thresholds for subclinical hypothyroidism were advocated—such as S. TSH levels of 2–2.5 mIU/L.[17,18] Depending on the definition used, prevalence among infertile women ranges from 16 to 20%.[12] Subclinical hypothyroidism is associated with decreased female fecundity[19,20] as a consequence of the raised LH levels and resulting anovulation.[21] However, some studies show no association between subclinical hypothyroidism and female infertility.[22,23] Subclinical hypothyroidism is associated with decreased ART success rates, and increased biochemical losses and miscarriages. Evidence shows a progressive rise in miscarriage rates with increasing

TSH levels, indicating that the risk correlates with the severity of thyroid dysfunction.[24]

Thyroid Autoimmunity

Thyroid autoimmunity refers to the presence of anti-thyroid peroxidase (anti-TPO) and/or anti-thyroglobulin (anti-TG) antibodies, which increase the risk of developing both subclinical and overt hypothyroidism.[25] A recent meta-analysis found that the *prevalence of thyroid autoantibody positivity in women with infertility is ~20%,* which is higher than typical estimates in the general population.[4]

Evidence consistently shows that women with thyroid autoantibodies often exhibit indicators of reduced ovarian reserve.[26-28] Anti-TPO and anti-TG antibodies are known to damage thyroid cells through complement activation and antibody-dependent cytotoxicity.[29] With TG and TPO antigens also identified in ovarian tissue (granulosa cells),[30,31] it is hypothesized that the same immune-mediated mechanisms could target ovarian cells, contributing to impaired follicular function and reduced ovarian reserve. Crossreactivity of TPOAbs with hCG in zona pellucida has also been proposed to be another mechanism of infertility.[32] This has been observed in the presence of high levels on anti-TPOAbs (>100 IU/mL) with S. TSH levels exceeding 2.5 mIU/L, while TGAbs alone appear to be less associated with adverse outcomes.[33]

Beyond their effect on ovarian reserve, thyroid autoimmunity (TAI) can disrupt local thyroid hormone production in the endometrium and placenta, affecting embryo implantation and placentation.[11,34] Systemic immune dysregulation, including altered T helper (Th)1/Th2/Th17 and natural killer (NK) cell activity, contributes to implantation failure and pregnancy loss.[35] Coexisting autoimmune disorders ([like systemic lupus erythematosus (SLE), Sjögren's, rheumatoid arthritis (RA), etc.] may amplify these effects, collectively increasing the risk of miscarriage, preterm delivery, and other adverse reproductive outcomes.[36]

Thyroid autoimmunity often coexists with polycystic ovarian syndrome (PCOS)[37] and endometriosis[38]—both established contributors to infertility—thereby further linking TAI to impaired reproductive outcomes. Further the rates of antiphospholipid antibody positivity are 3–4 times higher in women with thyroid autoimmunity compared to healthy controls. This results in higher chances of implantation failure as well as recurrent pregnancy losses.[39]

Subclinical and Overt Hyperthyroidism

The effect of hyperthyroidism on fertility is still poorly understood due to paucity of data.[40] Up to 5.8% women with hyperthyroidism may experience primary or secondary infertility[41] as a result of menstrual irregularities, often linked to hormonal imbalances such as elevated estradiol and androgens.[42]

It is most commonly caused by Graves' disease, an autoimmune disorder. It frequently coexists with other autoimmune disorders. The risk of miscarriages is significantly increased in the presence of untreated hyperthyroidism.[43]

SCREENING RECOMMENDATIONS

Recurrent Pregnancy Loss

In women with a history of recurrent pregnancy loss, several guidelines recommend to test S. TSH levels and anti-TPO antibodies in view of the well-documented association between thyroid dysfunction and miscarriages.

American Society of Reproductive Medicine (ASRM): Recommends screening for S. TSH in patients of RPL. Further screening for free T4 levels and anti-TPO antibodies is not routinely recommended in case of normal TSH levels. However, there is lack of consensus regarding whether to consider >4 mIU/L or >2.5 mIU/L as the cutoff for abnormal S. TSH levels.[44]

European Society for Human Reproduction and Endocrinology (ESHRE): Strongly recommends screening for S. TSH and anti-TPO antibodies in women with RPL.[45]

Royal College of Obstetricians and Gynecologists (RCOG): Recommends screening for thyroid function (S. TSH). Selective screening for anti-TPO antibodies should be done in women with RPL.

American College of Obstetricians and Gynecologists (ACOG)46 and American Thyroid Association (ATA):47 Both recommend screening of S. TSH for women with history of RPL (termed in the guidelines as "women with risk factor for thyroid disease"). Further anti-TPO testing is recommended only if there are abnormal TSH values, other autoimmune diseases or while monitoring at risk pregnant women.

Infertility and Assisted Reproductive Technology

American Society of Reproductive Medicine:[48] Recommends assessment of thyroid function (TSH ± free T4) as part of infertility evaluation, particularly before ART. It does not recommend routine anti-TPO testing in all infertile women; antibody testing may be considered selectively, especially in ART settings or abnormal TSH.

European Society for Human Reproduction and Endocrinology/Royal College of Obstetricians and Gynecologists: No specific guidelines regarding thyroid testing of infertile women.

American College of Obstetricians and Gynecologists:[46] Recommends TSH testing in women planning pregnancy or pregnant with risk factors; does not support universal screening in infertility. Routine anti-TPO testing is *not* recommended in euthyroid women.

American Thyroid Association:[47] Recommends *targeted (risk-based)* TSH testing in women planning pregnancy or undergoing fertility treatment; does not endorse universal screening of all infertile women. Does not recommend routine anti-TPO antibody testing in euthyroid infertile women; testing may be considered if TSH is abnormal or autoimmune disease is suspected **(Table 1)**.

TREATMENT GUIDELINES

Overt Hypothyroidism

Several organizations[45-49] universally recommend treatment of women with overt hypothyroidism with levothyroxine. Levothyroxine therapy should be promptly initiated with the target of restoring euthyroid status prior to conception (or as early in pregnancy as possible). This helps to improve fertility outcomes as well as prevention of miscarriages and other adverse obstetrics outcomes.

Subclinical Hypothyroidism

American Society of Reproductive Medicine recommends treatment of subclinical hypothyroidism in women attempting to conceive or undergoing ART, especially in TPO antibody positive. Target TSH values should be trimester-specific ranges.[48] ESHRE,[45] ATA,[47] and RCOG[49] recommend treatment of subclinical hypothyroidism in women with RPL and/or TPO antibody positivity, however, evidence for treatment of those with infertility without RPL is limited and treatment decisions are to be individualized.

Thyroid Autoimmunity

In euthyroid women who are anti-TPO antibody positive, it is important to make a distinction between those who have a history of RPL and those who do not.

History of RPL⁺: Routine therapy with levothyroxine is not recommended. During pregnancy close monitoring of thyroid function is advocated and prompt treatment should be initiated if subclinical hypothyroidism develops. Recent guidelines by prominent organizations bear this stance.[45,46] The shift from earlier recommendations (to consider low-dose LT4 supplementation)[47] is based on the evidence from recent randomized controlled trials (RCTs) (TABLET,[50] and T4LIFE[51]) that show no improvement in live birth rates with T4 supplementation.

No history of RPL: Routine therapy is not indicated and close monitoring of thyroid function in case of women at risk for thyroid disease should be carried out.

TABLE 1: Risk factors triggering thyroid testing in women planning pregnancy or undergoing fertility evaluation.

A. Universal medical risk factors	*B. Autoimmune and systemic disease risk factors*	*C. Reproductive risk factors*	*D. Pregnancy-related and obstetric risk factors*	*E. Triggers for anti-TPO antibody testing*
• Known thyroid disease (past or present) • Previous thyroid surgery or radioactive iodine therapy • History of postpartum thyroiditis • Goiter or thyroid nodules • Symptoms suggestive of thyroid dysfunction • Use of medications affecting thyroid function (e.g., amiodarone and lithium) • Family history of autoimmune thyroid disease (first-degree relative)	• Type 1 diabetes mellitus • Systemic lupus erythematosus • Rheumatoid arthritis • Celiac disease • Pernicious anemia • Other autoimmune disorders	• Infertility • Assisted reproductive technology (IVF/ICSI) • Recurrent pregnancy loss (RPL) • History of unexplained pregnancy loss • Premature ovarian insufficiency • Ovarian dysfunction	• History of miscarriage • History of preterm birth • Previous pregnancy complications suggestive of thyroid dysfunction • Maternal age >30–35 years • Obesity • Residence in areas of iodine deficiency or excess	• Abnormal TSH • Recurrent pregnancy loss • Known autoimmune disease • Prior pregnancy loss with normal fetal karyotype • Infertility with suspected immune contribution • Subclinical hypothyroidism
Practical testing implication				
• Perform *TSH* testing in all women with any risk factor listed in columns A–D • Add *anti-TPO antibody testing* when triggers in column E are present • Infertility or RPL alone justifies testing even in asymptomatic women • Routine population screening without risk factors is not recommended				

(ICSI: intracytoplasmic sperm injection; IVF: in-vitro fertilization; TPO: thyroid peroxidase; TSH: thyroid-stimulating hormone)

Hyperthyroidism[47]

All overt hyperthyroidisms must be treated with the intention to restore euthyroid state prior to conception. Propylthiouracil to be used in 1st trimester and methimazole in 2nd/3rd trimester. Beta-blockers can be used for symptom control. Radioactive iodine is to be avoided in women planning pregnancy. In case of subclinical hyperthyroidism, usually no treatment is required unless the S. TSH level is suppressed to <0.1 mIU/L and/or patient has symptoms/cardiac disease/osteoporosis, etc., close monitoring is necessary in pregnancy.

SPECIAL CONSIDERATIONS IN ASSISTED REPRODUCTIVE TECHNOLOGY

In ART cycles, where achieving a successful pregnancy is challenging and patient's investment—emotional, physical, and financial—is substantial, meticulous optimization of thyroid function becomes a crucial component of care. Both overt thyroid dysfunction and subclinical dysfunction/autoantibody positivity are implicated in altered ART outcomes.

Elevated TSH levels even in the upper limit of normal (particularly >2.5–4 mIU/L in TPO-positive women) have shown to impair implantation rates following IVF/ICSI.[52] Women with thyroid autoantibodies also show evidence of poor fertilization and low blastocyst formation rates.[53] Controlled ovarian stimulation (COS) elevates estradiol levels, leading to increased thyroxine-binding globulin and transient alterations in free thyroid hormone concentrations;[54] consequently, TSH may exert a more pronounced impact in fresh ART cycles, where COS-induced hormonal fluctuations are maximal, while frozen cycles appear less sensitive.[55]

Screening Recommendations

All women planned for ARTs should undergo a baseline S. TSH assessment prior to starting treatment, irrespective of symptoms given the narrow therapeutic window required for optimal implantation. Universal screening is supported by ASRM[56] as well as expert consensus review by ETA- and ESHRE-affiliated authors.[57] Anti-TPO antibody testing may be considered in those with recurrent implantation failure, unexplained infertility, and poor ovarian response in prior cycles and those with thyroid dysfunction.[57]

Treatment Targets

Most professional societies[47,56] agree that thyroid function should be optimized prior to initiation of ART, given that implantation and early pregnancy is highly sensitive to thyroid hormone availability. Recommended target is <2.5 mIU/L. COS-related estrogen surges may increase thyroxine-binding globulin (TBG) and alter thyroid tests; TSH trends, rather than isolated FT4 values, should guide management.

Hyperthyroidism is a contraindication to ART, biochemical euthyroid state must be achieved prior to initiation of therapy.[47]

CONCLUSION

Thyroid disorders are frequently present in women presenting with infertility and recurrent pregnancy loss, and their impact on reproductive outcomes is significant. As these endocrine disorders are easily recognizable and mostly treatable, focused attention to thyroid health offers the clinician a simple, yet effective way to improve clinical outcomes.

TAKE HOME POINTS

- Thyroid homeostasis is key to normal reproductive function influencing all stages—ovulation, endometrial receptivity, implantation, placentation, and early fetal development.
- Women with infertility and RPL exhibit a higher prevalence of thyroid dysfunction compared with the general population.
- Overt hypothyroidism and hyperthyroidism are associated with subfertility, ART failure, and miscarriage, and must be treated to achieve euthyroid state prior to conception.
- Subclinical hypothyroidism is associated with adverse reproductive and ART outcomes, particularly as TSH levels rise and in the presence of thyroid autoimmunity.
- Thyroid autoimmunity is linked to reduced ovarian reserve, implantation failure, and pregnancy loss through immune-mediated and endocrine mechanisms, even in euthyroid women.
- Routine levothyroxine therapy is not recommended in euthyroid, thyroid antibody-positive women, including those with RPL, based on evidence from recent randomized trials.
- In ART cycles, even mildly elevated TSH levels may negatively impact cycle success; baseline TSH assessment and pretreatment optimization are the standard-of-care.
- Hyperthyroidism is a contraindication to ART, and biochemical euthyroid state must be achieved before initiating treatment.
- Management of thyroid disorders in infertility and RPL should be individualized, evidence-based, and aligned with current international guidelines.
- Ongoing research into thyroid-immune-reproductive interactions is likely to further refine screening and treatment strategies in reproductive medicine.

REFERENCES

1. World Health Organization. 1 in 6 people globally affected by infertility: WHO [Internet]. Geneva: WHO; 2023.
2. El Hachem H, Crepaux V, May-Panloup P, Descamps P, Legendre G, Bouet PE. Recurrent pregnancy loss: current perspectives. Int J Women's Health. 2017;9:331-45.
3. Dong AC, Morgan J, Kane M, Stagnaro-Green A, Stephenson MD. Subclinical hypothyroidism and thyroid autoimmunity in recurrent pregnancy loss: a systematic review and meta-analysis. Fertil Steril. 2020;113(3):587-600.e1.
4. Huang Y, Xie B, Li J, Hang F, Hu Q, Jin Y, et al. Prevalence of thyroid autoantibody positivity in women with infertility: a systematic review and meta-analysis. BMC Women's Health. 2024;24:630.
5. Concepción-Zavaleta MJ, Coronado-Arroyo JC, Quiroz-Aldave JE, Concepción-Urteaga LA, Paz-Ibarra J. Thyroid dysfunction and female infertility. A comprehensive review. Diabetes Metab Syndr. 2023;17(11):102876.
6. Tan J, Yang YY, Yin Y, Xin Q, Ge XC. Research on the Impact of Thyroid Disorders on Reproductive Function: A Narrative Review. J Clin Med Res. 2025; 17(8):409-22.
7. Brown EDL, Obeng-Gyasi B, Hall JE, Shekhar S. The Thyroid Hormone Axis and Female Reproduction. Int J Mol Sci. 2023;24(12):9815.
8. Zhang C, Wang X, Wang Z, Niu W, Zhu B, Xia G. Effect of different culture systems and 3,5,3'-triiodothyronine/follicle-stimulating hormone on preantral follicle development in mice. PLoS One. 2013;8(4):e61947.
9. Kabodmehri R, Sharami SH, Sorouri ZZ, Gashti NG, Milani F, Chaypaz Z, et al. The relationship between thyroid function and ovarian reserve: a prospective cross-sectional study. Thyroid Res. 2021;14(1):22.
10. Colicchia M, Campagnolo L, Baldini E, Ulisse S, Valensise H, Moretti C. Molecular basis of thyrotropin and thyroid hormone action during implantation and early development. Hum Reprod Update. 2014;20(6):884-904.
11. Alexander EK, Pearce EN, Brent GA, Brown RS, Chen H, Dosiou C, et al. Thyroid Regulation and Dysfunction in the Pregnant Patient. In: Feingold KR, Anawalt B, Boyce A, Chrousos G, de Herder WW, Dhatariya K, et al., (Eds). Endotext. South Dartmouth (MA): MDText.com, Inc.; 2000-2025.
12. Dhillon-Smith RK, Tobias A, Smith PP, Middleton LJ, Sunner KK, Baker K, et al. The prevalence of thyroid dysfunction and autoimmunity in women with history of miscarriage or subfertility. J Clin Endocrinol Metab. 2020;105(8):2667-77.
13. Bahar A, Akha O, Kashi Z, Vesgari Z. Hyperprolactinemia in association with subclinical hypothyroidism. Caspian J Intern Med. 2011;2(2):229-33.
14. Yu Z, Feng X, Lin Z, Li X, Su S, Cheng H, et al. Thyroid hormone transport and metabolism are disturbed in the placental villi of miscarriage. Reprod Biol Endocrinol. 2023;21:108.
15. Repelaer van Driel-Delprat CC, van Dam EWCM, van de Ven PM, Aissa K, Ter Haar MK, Feenstra Y, et al. Thyroid function and IVF outcome for different indications of subfertility. Reprod Fertil. 2021;2(4):280-91.
16. Surks MI, Ortiz E, Daniels GH, Sawin CT, Col NF, Cobin RH, et al. Subclinical thyroid disease: scientific review and guidelines for diagnosis and management. JAMA. 2004;291:228-38.

17. Wartofsky L, Dickey RA. The evidence for a narrower thyrotropin reference range is compelling. J Clin Endocrinol Metab. 2005;90:5483-8.
18. Dayan CM, Saravanan P, Bayly G. Whose normal thyroid function is better—yours or mine? Lancet. 2002;360:353.
19. Feldthusen AD, Pedersen PL, Larsen J, Kristensen TT, Ellervik C, Kvetny J. Impaired fertility associated with subclinical hypothyroidism and thyroid autoimmunity: the Danish general suburban population study. J Pregnancy. 2015;2015:132718.
20. Hiraoka T, Wada-Hiraike O, Hirota Y, Hirata T, Koga K, Osuga Y, et al. The impact of elevated thyroid-stimulating hormone on female subfertility. Reprod Med Biol. 2016;15(2):121-6.
21. Al-Jaroudi D, Yassin S, Enezi NA, Kaddour O, Al-Badr A. Hypothyroidism among subfertile women. Clin Exp Obstet Gynecol. 2018;45(1):63-7.
22. Birjandi B, Ramezani Tehrani F, Amouzegar A, Tohidi M, Bidhendi Yarandi R, Azizi F. The association between subclinical hypothyroidism and TPOAb positivity with infertility in a population-based study: Tehran Thyroid Study (TTS). BMC Endocr Disord. 2021;21(1):108.
23. Jagun OE, Andu BA, Olawale OO. Subclinical hypothyroidism among infertile women at a tertiary hospital in South-West Nigeria. Afr Health Sci. 2022;22(2):444-50.
24. Maraka S, Ospina NM, O'Keeffe DT, Espinosa De Ycaza AE, Gionfriddo MR, Erwin PJ, et al. Subclinical Hypothyroidism in Pregnancy: A Systematic Review and Meta-Analysis. Thyroid. 2016;26(4):580-90.
25. Tańska K, Gietka-Czernel M, Glinicki P, Kozakowski J. Thyroid autoimmunity and its negative impact on female fertility and maternal pregnancy outcomes. Front Endocrinol. 2023;13:1049665.
26. Hsieh YT, Ho JYP. Thyroid autoimmunity is associated with higher risk of premature ovarian insufficiency—a nationwide Health Insurance Research Database study. Hum Reprod. 2021;36(6):1621-9.
27. Hasegawa Y, Kitahara Y, Osuka S, Tsukui Y, Kobayashi M, Iwase A. Effect of hypothyroidism and thyroid autoimmunity on the ovarian reserve: a systematic review and meta-analysis. Reprod Med Biol. 2021;21(1):e12427.
28. Korevaar TIM, Mínguez-Alarcón L, Messerlian C, de Poortere RA, Williams PL, Broeren MA, et al. Association of thyroid function and autoimmunity with ovarian reserve in women seeking infertility care. Thyroid. 2018;28(10):1349-58.
29. Bogusławska J, Godlewska M, Gajda E, Piekiełko-Witkowska A. Cellular and molecular basis of thyroid autoimmunity. Eur Thyroid J. 2022;11(1):e210024.
30. Aissiou S, Boucekkine N, Cunnane EM, Gashti NG, Oumeziane A, Kaci N. Expression of thyroid antigens in the female reproductive system. Afr J Reprod Health. 2024;28(9):145-52.
31. Monteleone P, Faviana P, Artini PG. Thyroid peroxidase identified in human granulosa cells: another piece to the thyroid–ovary puzzle? Gynecol Endocrinol. 2017;33(7):574-6.
32. Twig G, Shina A, Amital H, Shoenfeld Y. Pathogenesis of infertility and recurrent pregnancy loss in thyroid autoimmunity. J Autoimmun. 2012;38(2-3):J275-81.
33. Zhang S, Wang Y, Li X, Liu H, Yang Y, Chen Q, et al. Relationship between thyroid antibody levels and ovarian reserve function in infertile Chinese women with normal thyroid-stimulating hormone. J Ovarian Res. 2023;16:100.

34. Rahnama R, Mahmoudi AR, Kazemnejad S, Salehi M, Ghahiri A, Soltanghoraee H, et al. Thyroid peroxidase in human endometrium and placenta: A potential target for anti-TPO antibodies. Clin Exp Med. 2021;21(1):79-88.
35. Saito S, Nakashima A, Shima T, Ito M. Th1/Th2/Th17 and regulatory T-cell paradigm in pregnancy. Am J Reprod Immunol. 2010;63(6):601-10.
36. Szeliga A, Calik-Ksepka A, Maciejewska-Jeske M, Grymowicz M, Smolarczyk K, Kostrzak A, et al. Autoimmune diseases in patients with premature ovarian insufficiency—our current state of knowledge. Int J Mol Sci. 2021;22(5):2594.
37. Romitti M, Fabris VC, Ziegelmann PK, Maia AL, Spritzer PM. Association between PCOS and autoimmune thyroid disease: a systematic review and meta-analysis. Endocr Connect. 2018;7(11):1158-67.
38. Eisenberg VH, Zolti M, Soriano D. Is there an association between autoimmunity and endometriosis? Autoimmun Rev. 2012;11:806-14.
39. Lu D, Song Z, Gao Y, Zhang J, Guo X. Patients with Autoimmune Thyroid Diseases Have Higher Prevalence of Positive Antiphospholipid Antibodies: A Systematic Review and Meta-Analysis. Int J Endocrinol. 2022;2022:8271951.
40. Andersen SL, Olsen J, Wu CS, Laurberg P. Spontaneous abortion, stillbirth and hyperthyroidism: a Danish population-based study. Eur Thyroid J. 2014;3(3):164-72.
41. Mintziori G, Kita M, Duntas L, Goulis DG. Consequences of hyperthyroidism in male and female fertility: pathophysiology and current management. J Endocrinol Invest. 2016;39(8):849-53.
42. Southren AL, Olivo J, Gordon GG, Vittek J, Brener J, Rafii F. The conversion of androgens to estrogens in hyperthyroidism. J Clin Endocrinol Metab. 1974;38(2):207-14.
43. Joshi JV, Bhandarkar SD, Chadha M, Balaiah D, Shah R. Menstrual irregularities and lactation failure may precede thyroid dysfunction or goitre. J Postgrad Med. 1993;39(3):137-41.
44. Practice Committee of the American Society for Reproductive Medicine. Evaluation and treatment of recurrent pregnancy loss: a committee opinion. Fertil Steril. 2012;98(5):1103-11.
45. Bender Atik R, Christiansen OB, Elson J, Kolte AM, Lewis S, Middeldorp S, et al. ESHRE guideline: recurrent pregnancy loss: an update in 2022. Hum Reprod Open. 2023;2023(1):hoad002.
46. American College of Obstetricians and Gynecologists. Thyroid disease in pregnancy. Practice Bulletin No. 228. Obstet Gynecol. 2020;136(6):e1-18.
47. Alexander EK, Pearce EN, Brent GA, Brown RS, Chen H, Dosiou C, et al. 2017 guidelines of the American Thyroid Association for the diagnosis and management of thyroid disease during pregnancy and the postpartum. Thyroid. 2017;27(3):315-89.
48. Penzias A, Amato P, Anderson J, Bendikson K, Gracia C, Falcone T, et al.; Practice Committee of the American Society for Reproductive Medicine; ASRM Subclinical Hypothyroidism Guideline Task Force. Subclinical hypothyroidism in the infertile female population: a guideline. Fertil Steril. 2024;121(5):765-82.
49. Chan SY, Marsh MS, Gilbert J, Boelaert K, Evans C, Dhillon Smith R; on behalf of the Royal College of Obstetricians and Gynaecologists. Management of thyroid disorders in pregnancy: Green top Guideline No. 76. BJOG. 2025;132:e130-61.

50. Dhillon Smith RK, Middleton LJ, Sunner KK, Smith PP, Baker K, Farrell-Carver S, et al. Levothyroxine to increase live births in euthyroid women with thyroid antibodies trying to conceive: the TABLET randomized controlled trial. BMJ. 2019;366:l4896.
51. van Dijk M, van Dijk R, Timmers T, van Montfoort AP, Mol BW, van der Veen F, et al. Levothyroxine in euthyroid women with recurrent pregnancy loss and positive TPO Ab: the T4LIFE randomized controlled trial. Fertil Steril. 2022;118(5):938-47.
52. Zhou P, Yao Q, Zhao Q, Yang L, Yu Y, Xie J, et al. IVF/ICSI outcomes of euthyroid infertile women with thyroid autoimmunity: does treatment with aspirin plus prednisone matter? BMC Pregnancy Childbirth. 2022;22:263.
53. Busnelli A, Paffoni A, Fedele L, Somigliana E. The impact of thyroid autoimmunity on IVF/ICSI outcome: a systematic review and meta-analysis. Hum Reprod Update. 2016;22(6):775-90. Erratum in: Hum Reprod Update. 2016;22(6):793-4.
54. Gracia CR, Morse CB, Chan G, Schilling S, Prewitt M, Sammel MD, et al. Thyroid function during controlled ovarian hyperstimulation as part of in vitro fertilization. J Clin Endocrinol Metab. 2012;97(2):545-54.
55. Li D, Hu S, Meng X, Yu X. Changes in thyroid function during controlled ovarian hyperstimulation (COH) and its impact on assisted reproduction technology (ART) outcomes: a systematic review and meta-analysis. J Assist Reprod Genet. 2021;38(9):2227-35.
56. Practice Committee of the American Society for Reproductive Medicine. Subclinical hypothyroidism in the infertile female population: a guideline. Fertil Steril. 2015;104(3):545-53.
57. Poppe K, Velkeniers B, Glinoer D, et al. Thyroid disorders in infertile women. Hum Reprod Update. 2021;27(3):418-29.

CHAPTER 8

Myths and Realities (Thyroid and Pregnancy)

Zubin Sheriar

Myth: Women with hypothyroidism cannot become pregnant.

Fact: Conception is possible for women with hypothyroidism, provided the condition is properly treated and monitored. When left unmanaged, however, hypothyroidism can make it harder to conceive.

Myth: Normal thyroid-stimulating hormone (TSH) values on a laboratory report rule out thyroid problems in pregnancy.

Fact: Standard TSH ranges for nonpregnant women are 0.5–5.0 mIU/L. During pregnancy, trimester-specific ranges must be used instead:

- *First trimester:* 0.6–3.4 mU/L
- *Second trimester:* 0.37–3.6 mU/L
- *Third trimester:* 0.38–4.0 mU/L

Therefore, interpreting TSH without considering the trimester may be misleading.

Myth: Thyroid medication should be discontinued during pregnancy.

Fact: Maintaining thyroid hormone treatment during pregnancy is crucial. Stopping medication can result in uncontrolled thyroid levels and potential complications.

Myth: Hyperemesis gravidarum causes hyperthyroidism.

Fact: Severe vomiting in pregnancy is linked to very high human chorionic gonadotropin (hCG) levels, which can temporarily elevate thyroid hormones. This short-lived hyperthyroidism requires careful evaluation through history, examination, and laboratory tests to distinguish it from true thyroid disease.

Myth: Thyroid disorders are the main cause of weight gain.

Fact: Although the thyroid regulates metabolism, significant weight gain from untreated hypothyroidism is uncommon. In severe cases, added weight often comes from fluid retention—not fat—and resolves once thyroid hormone levels are corrected.

Myth: Breastfeeding is unsafe while taking thyroid medication.

Fact: Only a minimal amount of thyroid hormone passes into breast milk, making these medications safe to use during breastfeeding.

Myth: Pregnant women need large amounts of iodine to keep the thyroid functioning.

Fact: Iodine is vital for hormone production, and pregnancy increases the daily requirement to about *250 μg*. However, excessive iodine—especially from supplements like seaweed—can actually trigger thyroid problems.

Myth: Thyroid problems during pregnancy require a special diet.

Fact: Beyond ensuring adequate iodine intake, pregnant women with thyroid disorders generally only need the same balanced, and nutritious diet recommended for all pregnancies.

Myth: Soy products are harmful for thyroid conditions.

Fact: Soy does not damage the thyroid but can reduce absorption of thyroid medication. It is best not to take your medication with soy-rich meals.

Myth: Going gluten-free can cure Hashimoto's thyroiditis or prevent thyroid disease in pregnancy.

Fact: Hashimoto's is the leading cause of hypothyroidism, and eliminating gluten does *not* reverse it. While people with celiac disease must avoid gluten—and celiac disease is somewhat more common in those with Hashimoto's—there is no evidence that gluten-free eating prevents thyroid disorders.

Index

Page numbers followed by *f* refer to figure and *t* refer to table.

U

V

W